A COMPREHENSIVE GUIDE TO HEALTHCARE QUALITY

Asaad bin Abdulrahman Abduljawad,
CHQ, M.P.H, Dr.PH, FAIHQ

A Comprehensive Guide to Healthcare Quality

Authored by Dr. Asaad Bin Abdulrahman Abduljawad, MPH, DrPH
Edmond, Oklahoma

Library of Congress Control Number

(LCCN): 2024926656

ISBN: 979-8-218-57650-9

Dedication

To the souls of my beloved parents, whose continuous prayers to Allah Almighty for my success guided and blessed me through every step of my life. Their sacrifices in providing me with the best education, enrolling me in the best schools, and their relentless encouragement throughout my academic journey shaped who I am today.

To my country, the holy land of the Kingdom of Saudi Arabia, to leaders, policymakers, healthcare professionals, providers, and students.

And finally, to my wonderful children Abdulrahman and his siblings, my family, whose love and joy inspired me.

With deepest gratitude,

Dr. Asaad bin Abdulrahman Abduljawad

Acknowledgements

I would like to extend my deepest gratitude to His Excellency Professor A. F. Al-Assaf, MD, MPH, Distinguished Presidential and Regents' Professor Emeritus at the University of Oklahoma and Executive Director of the American Institute for Healthcare Quality. His exceptional mentorship, unwavering guidance, and invaluable support have been instrumental in the completion of this book.

Professor Al-Assaf's expertise in public health, medical quality, and patient safety has profoundly influenced my work. His meticulous review of all the chapters, insightful suggestions, and assistance in refining the content have significantly enhanced the quality of this book. The idea of writing this book was inspired by his visionary approach, and I am honored to follow in his footsteps.

Thank you, Professor Al-Assaf, for your dedication and for being a pillar of knowledge and inspiration.

Contents

Kingdom of Saudi Arabia
Saudi Health Council
Saudi Central Board for Accreditation
of Healthcare Institutions

CBAHI

المملكة العربية السعودية
المجلس الصحي السعودي
المركز السعودي لاعتماد المنشآت الصحية
(٤٥٦)

Foreword

It is with great pleasure that I endorse "A Comprehensive Guide to Healthcare Quality" authored by H.E. Dr. Asaad bin Abdulrahman Abduljawad. This book is a testament to the profound commitment to excellence in healthcare that we strive for at the Saudi Central Board for Accreditation of Healthcare Institutions (CBAHI).

In an era where the quality of healthcare services is paramount, this comprehensive guide serves as an invaluable resource for healthcare students, healthcare professionals, administrators, and policymakers. Dr. Abduljawad's extensive experience and deep understanding of healthcare quality and patient safety are evident throughout the pages of this book. His ability to distill complex concepts into practical, actionable strategies makes this work an essential tool for anyone dedicated to improving healthcare outcomes.

The topics covered in this book, ranging from strategic planning, risk management, and patient safety to performance measures and regulatory compliance, provide a holistic view of the multifaceted nature of healthcare quality. Each chapter is meticulously crafted to offer insights and guidance that are both relevant and timely, reflecting the latest advancements and best practices in the field.

As the Director General of CBAHI, I have witnessed firsthand the transformative impact that a focus on quality can have on healthcare institutions. This book not only underscores the importance of quality and safety but also equips readers with the knowledge and tools necessary to drive continuous improvement in their organizations.

I commend Dr. Abduljawad for his dedication in educating, training, and professionally advancing healthcare quality and patient safety in the Kingdom of Saudi Arabia, and for providing this comprehensive guide that will undoubtedly serve as a cornerstone for healthcare professionals striving for excellence. It is my hope that this book will inspire and empower its readers to achieve the highest standards of care, ultimately benefiting patients and communities across the globe.

Sincerely,

Dr. Salem bin Abdullah Al-Wahabi
Director General of the Saudi Central Board for Accreditation of Healthcare Institutions (CBAHI)

Preface

I cannot start out talking about quality without referring to a true leader's quote Prophet Mohammed PBUH says: "Verily, GOD almighty loves that when anyone of you does a job, he should perfect it.". The pursuit of healthcare quality is a journey that requires dedication, knowledge, and a commitment to continuous improvement. Over the years, I have had the privilege of teaching medical and public health students, graduate students at the University of Oklahoma Health Sciences Center (OUHSC), and undergraduate students at Umm Al-Qura University. Additionally, I have taught medical residents and fellows in the Saudi Board of Preventive Medicine, and served as an item writer for the Saudi Medical Licensing Exam and Professional Licensing Exams at the Saudi Commission for Healthcare Specialties.

My professional journey has included working with the Veteran Affairs, Integris Health System, and Mercy Hospitals in Oklahoma during my Master's and doctoral studies. I completed my postdoctoral fellowship in healthcare quality and patient safety with Baylor, Texas A&M in Dallas, and earned certifications from the STEEEP Academy at Baylor Scott & White. I also became a Lean Leader from Integris Health System in Oklahoma City, obtained a Green Belt in Healthcare Lean Six Sigma from the College of Engineering at the University of Michigan, Ann Arbor, and received a CHQ certificate from the University of Oklahoma. Additionally, I work as a consultant with AGI Consulting, USA, and completed executive leadership training at the Harvard School of Public Health in Boston, MA.

I have had the honor of serving as the Dean of the College of Health Sciences at Umm Al-Qura University in Saudi Arabia and the Dean of International Affairs at the American Institute for Healthcare Quality (AIHQ) in the United States of America. My work has extended internationally, consulting with Accreditation Kazakhstan and heading the training committee at the Central Asian Council. Additionally, I have worked as a trainer with the Saudi Patient Safety Center and as an executive advisor at the Saudi Electronic University and the Saudi Commission for Healthcare Specialties.

These diverse experiences have provided me with a comprehensive understanding of the challenges and opportunities in healthcare quality. It is this wealth of knowledge and practical experience that I aim to share through this book. "A Comprehensive Guide to Healthcare Quality" is designed as an outline for professionals who need time to study and remember the key points from my lectures. This book is dedicated to providing clear applications and simplified examples to effectively convey key concepts, ensuring that my students and readers can gain enjoyment and interest in the subject.

Introduction

Ensuring high standards of healthcare quality is both a challenge and a necessity in today's complex and dynamic healthcare environment. This book, "A Comprehensive Guide to Healthcare Quality," is designed to serve as a valuable resource for healthcare professionals, administrators, and students who are passionate about enhancing the quality of care provided to patients.

Healthcare quality encompasses a wide range of concepts, from the structural aspects of healthcare facilities to the intricate details of patient safety and performance measurement. Each chapter in this book addresses a critical component of healthcare quality, providing readers with a thorough understanding of the principles and practices that drive excellence in this field.

Chapter Outline

Chapter 1: Hospitals and Healthcare Facilities

This chapter introduces the different types of healthcare institutions, including long-term care, primary care, ambulatory care, home health, and behavioral health. It also discusses the levels of care: primary, secondary, tertiary, and quaternary.

Chapter 2: Leadership

Explores the comparison between leadership and management, examining various types and styles of leadership that are essential in healthcare settings.

Chapter 3: Quality Concepts and Gurus

Traces the evolution of quality and healthcare quality, highlighting the contributions of key figures and the development of quality concepts over time.

Chapter 4: Strategic Planning

Provides an overview of the basics of healthcare strategic planning, including SWOT analysis, mission, vision, values, and examples. It also discusses organizational charts and the roles within healthcare organizations.

Chapter 5: Health Directives

Examines the importance of policies, procedures, pathways, guidelines, protocols, algorithms, and standard operating procedures (SOPs) in maintaining healthcare quality.

Chapter 6: Performance Measures

Focuses on measuring quality through Key Performance Indicators (KPIs), providing examples from various medical disciplines.

Chapter 7: Patient Safety

Addresses patient safety, discussing seminal works such as the Institute of Medicine's "Crossing the Quality Chasm" and "To Err is Human." It also covers Reason's Swiss Cheese Model, types of clinical errors, Root Cause Analysis (RCA), and Failure Modes and Effects Analysis (FMEA).

Chapter 8: Quality Tools

Introduces various tools used in quality improvement initiatives, including brainstorming, multi-voting, process mapping, Pareto charts, histograms, bar charts, pie charts, run charts, and the concepts of common cause and special cause variation.

Chapter 9: Quantitative Analysis

Covers essential statistical methods such as sampling, mean, mode, median, variance, standard deviation, central tendency, normal distribution, t-tests, ANOVA, and linear regression. These methods are crucial for analyzing healthcare data and supporting evidence-based decision-making.

Chapter 10: Quality and Process Improvement

Discusses change management and quality improvement methodologies such as PDCA (Plan-Do-Check-Act), FOCUS PDCA, Lean, and Six Sigma.

Chapter 11: Team Management

Explores the dynamics of groups and team building, outlining the steps necessary to create and lead effective teams in healthcare settings.

Chapter 12: Healthcare Regulatory and Compliance

Reviews the processes of licensing, certification, credentialing, privileging, and accreditation, along with the roles of accrediting bodies in ensuring healthcare quality.

Chapter 13: Health Information Management

Covers the management of electronic medical records (EMR) and electronic health records (EHR), the structure of computers, and the concepts of sensitivity, specificity, and the 2x2 contingency table.

Chapter 14: Risk Management

Provides an introduction to the basics of risk management, emphasizing the identification, assessment, and mitigation of risks in healthcare to ensure the safety and well-being of patients and staff.

This book is designed to be a comprehensive resource that equips readers with the knowledge and skills necessary to excel in the field of healthcare quality. It is my hope that this guide will serve as a valuable tool for those dedicated to improving healthcare systems and outcomes.

Truly,
Dr. Asaad bin Abdulrahman Abduljawad

Chapter 1

Hospital and Healthcare Facility Types

Hospital Types are classified:

By Ownership

Hospitals can be categorized by ownership into three main types: non-profit, for-profit, and government-owned. Non-profit hospitals, which make up nearly half of all hospitals in the U.S., reinvest their earnings into the hospital's services and community programs. For-profit hospitals, constituting about 36.1%, distribute profits to shareholders and are often part of larger healthcare chains. Government-owned hospitals, which account for approximately 14.7%, are funded and operated by local, state, or federal governments and often serve specific populations such as veterans or low-income individuals (Welch et al., 2023).

Differences Between For-Profit and Non-Profit Hospitals

Ownership and Governance

For-profit hospitals are typically owned by private entities or corporations, which may be publicly traded on the stock market. These hospitals are managed with the primary goal of generating profits for shareholders (Popowitz, 2023). In contrast, non-profit hospitals are often established by charitable organizations, religious groups, or community initiatives. They are governed by a board of trustees and are required to reinvest any surplus revenue back into the hospital's operations and community services (Zheng, 2023).

Financial Structure

The financial structures of for-profit and non-profit hospitals differ significantly. For-profit hospitals prioritize revenue generation and profitability. They rely on investments, patient fees, and insurance reimbursements to fund their operations (Popowitz, 2023). Non-profit hospitals, on the other hand, benefit from tax exemptions at the federal, state, and local levels. They also rely heavily on philanthropic donations and government grants to support their mission of providing accessible healthcare (Zheng, 2023).

Resource Allocation

Resource allocation in for-profit hospitals is often influenced by the need to generate profits. These hospitals may prioritize services that are more profitable, such as elective surgeries and advanced diagnostic procedures, and invest in marketing and advertising to attract more patients (Popowitz, 2023). Non-profit hospitals, however, focus on providing a broader range of community-oriented services, including emergency psychiatric care, addiction recovery programs, and trauma wards, which may not be as profitable but are essential for community health (Zheng, 2023).

Tax Status

One of the most significant differences between for-profit and non-profit hospitals is their tax status. For-profit hospitals are required to pay property and income taxes, which can impact their financial strategies and resource allocation (Mount Sinai, 2014). Non-profit hospitals are exempt from these taxes, allowing them to allocate more resources towards patient care and community services (Mount Sinai, 2014).

Access to Capital

For-profit hospitals have greater access to capital through investments from shareholders and the ability to raise funds through the stock market. This financial flexibility allows them to invest in new technologies and expand their services more readily (Health Leaders, 2019). Non-profit hospitals, while benefiting from tax exemptions and donations, may face challenges in raising capital and often rely on fundraising efforts and grants to finance their operations and improvements (Health Leaders, 2019).

Community Benefits

Non-profit hospitals are mandated to provide community benefits as part of their tax-exempt status. This includes offering free or reduced-cost care to low-income patients, conducting community health assessments, and implementing programs to address public health needs (Healthcare Dive, 2017). For-profit hospitals, while also providing high-quality care, are not required to offer the same level of community benefits and may focus more on services that enhance profitability (Healthcare Dive, 2017).

By Organizational Affiliation

Hospitals can also be classified based on their organizational affiliation. This includes independent hospitals, which operate on their own, and those that are part of larger health systems or networks. Health systems can be multi-hospital systems or single diversified hospital systems, which include one hospital and multiple pre- or post-acute care organizations (American Hospital Association, 2021). Affiliations can also include clinical affiliations, regional collaboratives, accountable care organizations (ACOs), and joint ventures (Texas Healthcare Trustees, 2017).

By Services

Hospitals are often categorized by the range of services they provide. General hospitals offer a wide array of services including emergency care, surgery, and obstetrics. Specialty hospitals focus on specific areas such as cardiac care, orthopedics, or cancer treatment (Liu et al., 2018). Community hospitals, which are the most common, provide general medical and surgical care for acute conditions (Liu et al., 2018).

By Population Served and Location

Hospitals can be classified based on the population they serve and their location. Urban hospitals are typically larger and offer a wider range of services compared to rural hospitals, which may have fewer resources and serve smaller populations (American Hospital Association, 2024). Community hospitals serve the general public, while federal hospitals serve specific groups such as military personnel and veterans (American Hospital Association, 2024).

By Size

Hospitals are often categorized by their size, which is typically measured by the number of beds. Small hospitals have fewer than 100 beds, medium hospitals have between 100 and 499 beds, and large hospitals have 500 or more beds (Gallagher Healthcare, 2018). The size of a hospital can influence the range of services it provides and its capacity to handle complex medical cases (Definitive Healthcare, 2024).

By Teaching Status

Hospitals can be classified as major teaching, minor teaching, or non-teaching hospitals. Major teaching hospitals are affiliated with medical schools and have a significant number of medical residents and fellows (Burke et al., 2017). Minor teaching hospitals have fewer residents and are often affiliated with smaller medical schools. Non-teaching hospitals do not have residency programs and focus primarily on providing patient care (Burke et al., 2017).

By Level of Care

Hospitals are also categorized by the level of care they provide, which includes primary, secondary, tertiary, and quaternary care. Primary care involves general health services provided by primary care physicians. Secondary care includes specialized services provided by specialists upon referral from a primary care provider. Tertiary care involves highly specialized medical care, often provided in large hospitals or academic medical centers, and includes services such as advanced surgery and cancer treatment. Quaternary care is an extension of tertiary care and includes experimental treatments and procedures (Torrey, 2024).

Differences Between Primary, Secondary, Tertiary, and Quaternary Healthcare Organizations

Primary Healthcare Organizations:

Primary healthcare organizations serve as the first point of contact for individuals within the healthcare system. They provide comprehensive, accessible, community-based care that meets the majority of an individual's health needs. Primary care includes prevention, wellness, and treatment for common illnesses and conditions (Starfield, 1998). Examples of primary healthcare organizations include:

Community Health Centers: These centers provide primary care services to underserved populations, focusing on preventive care and chronic disease management (Shi & Singh, 2022).

Family Medicine Practices: These practices offer continuous and comprehensive care for individuals and families across all ages, genders, diseases, and parts of the body (Saultz, 2000).

Secondary Healthcare Organizations:

Secondary healthcare organizations provide specialized medical services typically upon referral from a primary care provider. These services are more focused and involve the expertise of specialists who have advanced training in specific areas of medicine (Forrest, 2003). **Examples of secondary healthcare organizations include:**

Cardiology Clinics: These clinics specialize in diagnosing and treating heart conditions and diseases, often requiring referrals from primary care physicians (Forrest, 2003).

Orthopedic Centers: These centers focus on the diagnosis, treatment, and rehabilitation of musculoskeletal conditions, including bones, joints, ligaments, tendons, and muscles (Forrest, 2003).

Tertiary Healthcare Organizations

Tertiary healthcare organizations provide highly specialized care, often involving advanced and complex procedures and treatments. These organizations are typically large hospitals or academic medical centers that offer a wide range of specialized services (Garg et al., 2014). Examples of tertiary healthcare organizations include:

University Hospitals: These hospitals are affiliated with medical schools and provide advanced medical care, including specialized surgeries and treatments (Garg et al., 2014).

Cancer Treatment Centers: These centers offer comprehensive cancer care, including chemotherapy, radiation therapy, and surgical oncology (Garg et al., 2014).

Quaternary Healthcare Organizations

Quaternary healthcare organizations represent an extension of tertiary care, providing even more specialized and experimental treatments. These organizations often engage in cutting-edge research and offer treatments that are not widely available (Torrey, 2024). Examples of quaternary healthcare organizations include transplant centers and,

Experimental Medicine Centers: These centers conduct clinical trials and offer experimental treatments for various conditions, often involving new drugs or therapies (Torrey, 2024).

Advanced Neurosurgery Units: These units provide highly specialized neurosurgical procedures that are not commonly performed in other hospitals (Torrey, 2024).

Differences Between Acute and Chronic Care Services and Hospitals

Acute Care Services and Hospitals

Acute care services are designed to provide immediate and short-term treatment for severe or urgent medical conditions. These services are typically delivered in acute care hospitals, which are equipped to handle emergencies, surgeries, and other critical care needs (Geriatric Academy, 2024). Acute care hospitals focus on stabilizing patients and addressing life-threatening conditions, with the goal of discharging patients as soon as they are medically stable (Medical News Today, 2024).

Examples of acute care services include:

- Emergency Departments: These units provide immediate care for acute illnesses and injuries, such as heart attacks, strokes, and trauma from accidents (Geriatric Academy, 2024).
- Intensive Care Units (ICUs): These units offer specialized care for critically ill patients who require constant monitoring and advanced medical interventions (Medical News Today, 2024).

Chronic Care Services and Hospitals

Chronic care services are aimed at managing long-term health conditions that require ongoing medical attention and support. These services are often provided in chronic care hospitals or long-term care facilities, which cater to patients with persistent health issues that cannot be fully cured but can be managed over time (Verywell Health, 2023). Chronic care focuses on improving the quality of life for patients through continuous treatment, rehabilitation, and support (National Council on Aging, 2024).

Examples of chronic care services include:

- Diabetes Management Programs: These programs provide ongoing care and education to help patients manage their diabetes and prevent complications (Verywell Health, 2023).

- Chronic Obstructive Pulmonary Disease (COPD) Clinics: These clinics offer specialized care for patients with chronic respiratory conditions, focusing on symptom management and improving lung function (National Council on Aging, 2024).

Inpatient vs. Outpatient Services

Outpatient Care

Outpatient care, also known as ambulatory care, refers to medical services provided without requiring an overnight stay in a hospital or other inpatient facility. This type of care can encompass a wide range of services, from primary care to specialized treatments. Primary care, which is often delivered in an outpatient setting, includes routine check-ups, preventive care, and management of chronic conditions (Shi & Singh, 2022). Recently, outpatient care has expanded to include more specialized services such as minor surgeries, diagnostic tests, and certain types of therapy (American Hospital Association, 2021). Insurance companies often encourage outpatient care to reduce costs and limit inpatient care to the sickest patients for the shortest time possible (Healthline, 2023).

Inpatient Care

Inpatient care involves an overnight stay in a hospital or other healthcare facility. This type of care is typically required for more severe or complex medical conditions that necessitate close monitoring and intensive treatment. Examples of inpatient care include major surgeries, childbirth, and treatment for serious illnesses such as heart attacks or strokes (Geriatric Academy, 2024). Inpatient care is generally more expensive due to the extended use of hospital resources, including room and board, nursing care, and specialized medical equipment (Medical News Today, 2024).

Ambulatory Care

Ambulatory care is a broad term that encompasses all types of healthcare services provided to patients who are not admitted to a hospital. This includes primary care, as well as various subspecialties that do not require an overnight stay. Ambulatory care settings can range from doctor's offices and clinics to outpatient surgery centers and urgent care facilities (American Hospital Association, 2021). The focus of ambulatory care is on providing convenient, accessible, and cost-effective healthcare services (Shi & Singh, 2022).

Primary Care

Primary care is a field of medicine that serves as the first point of contact for patients within the healthcare system. It involves comprehensive and continuous care for individuals and families, addressing a wide range of health issues and coordinating all specialty care (Starfield, 1998). Primary care physicians play a crucial role in managing overall patient health, providing preventive care, diagnosing and treating common illnesses, and referring patients to specialists when necessary (Saultz, 2000).

Hospital Characteristics

Inpatient Capacity

Inpatient capacity refers to the number of beds available in a hospital for patients who require overnight stays. This capacity is a critical factor in determining a hospital's ability to handle patient volume and provide adequate care during peak times. Hospitals with higher inpatient capacity can accommodate more patients and offer a wider range of services, including intensive care and specialized treatments (American Hospital Association, 2021).

Licensed

Hospitals must be licensed by the state in which they operate. Licensing ensures that hospitals meet specific standards of care and safety as mandated by state health departments. The licensing process typically involves regular inspections and compliance with state regulations regarding staffing, facilities, and patient care protocols (Centers for Medicare & Medicaid Services, 2024).

Accredited

Accreditation is a voluntary process that hospitals undergo to demonstrate their commitment to meeting high standards of care and operational excellence. Accredited hospitals are evaluated by independent organizations such as The Joint Commission, which assesses various aspects of hospital operations, including patient safety, quality of care, and organizational management (The Joint Commission, 2024). Accreditation can enhance a hospital's reputation and ensure compliance with federal healthcare regulations (Centers for Medicare & Medicaid Services, 2024).

A Governing Body and a CEO

Hospitals are typically overseen by a governing body, such as a board of trustees, which is responsible for setting policies and ensuring the hospital's financial and operational stability. The Chief Executive Officer (CEO) is appointed by the governing body and is responsible for the day-to-day management of the hospital. The CEO's duties include strategic planning, resource allocation, and ensuring compliance with healthcare regulations (American Hospital Association, 2021).

Pharmacy

A hospital pharmacy is an integral part of the healthcare system, providing medications and pharmaceutical care to inpatients and outpatients. Hospital pharmacies are responsible for the procurement, storage, and dispensing of medications, as well as ensuring the safe and effective use of pharmaceuticals. Pharmacists in hospital settings also play a crucial role in patient education and medication management (American Society of Health-System Pharmacists, 2023).

Food Services

Hospital food services are essential for providing nutritious meals to patients, staff, and visitors. These services must adhere to dietary guidelines and accommodate various dietary restrictions and preferences. Proper nutrition is vital for patient recovery and overall health, making food services a critical component of hospital operations (Academy of Nutrition and Dietetics, 2023).

Medical Records Capacity

The capacity to manage medical records efficiently is crucial for hospital operations. Medical records include patient histories, treatment plans, and diagnostic information. Hospitals must maintain accurate and secure records to ensure continuity of care, support clinical decision-making, and comply with legal and regulatory requirements. The transition to electronic health records (EHRs) has improved the accessibility and management of medical records, enhancing the quality of care provided (HealthIT.gov, 2023).

Governing Body of a Hospital:

Also Known as the Board of Trustees, is the governing body of a hospital, commonly referred to as the board of trustees, plays a crucial role in overseeing the hospital's operations and strategic direction. This body is responsible for ensuring that the hospital adheres to its mission and long-term vision, which includes setting policies, defining strategic goals, and making high-level decisions that impact the overall functioning of the hospital (BoardEffect, 2018).

Responsibilities for Hospital Operations and Strategy

The board of trustees is tasked with several key responsibilities that are essential for the effective governance of the hospital. These responsibilities include:

Defining Strategic Goals: The board sets the long-term strategic goals for the hospital, which guide its mission and vision. This involves identifying priorities, allocating resources, and ensuring that the hospital's activities align with its strategic objectives (Boardable, 2024).

Hiring and Overseeing the CEO: One of the primary duties of the board is to hire and oversee the Chief Executive Officer (CEO). The board monitors the CEO's performance, provides guidance, and ensures that the CEO's actions are in line with the hospital's strategic goals (BoardEffect, 2018).

Ensuring Quality of Care: The board is responsible for ensuring that the hospital provides high-quality patient care. This includes monitoring patient outcomes, implementing quality improvement initiatives, and ensuring compliance with healthcare regulations and standards (Boardable, 2024).

Financial Oversight: The board oversees the hospital's financial health, ensuring that it remains financially sustainable. This involves approving budgets, monitoring financial performance, and making decisions about major capital investments (BoardEffect, 2018).

Community Representation: The board serves as a representative of the hospital within the community. It engages with community stakeholders, addresses community health needs, and ensures that the hospital's services are accessible and responsive to the community it serves (Boardable, 2024).

Types of Organizational Charts

Vertical Organizational Chart

A vertical organizational chart, also known as a hierarchical chart, is the most commonly used type of organizational structure. In this model, power is concentrated at the top, with each employee reporting to a superior above them. This structure creates a clear chain of command and delineates specific duties for each employee, ensuring accountability and clarity in roles (Venngage, 2023).

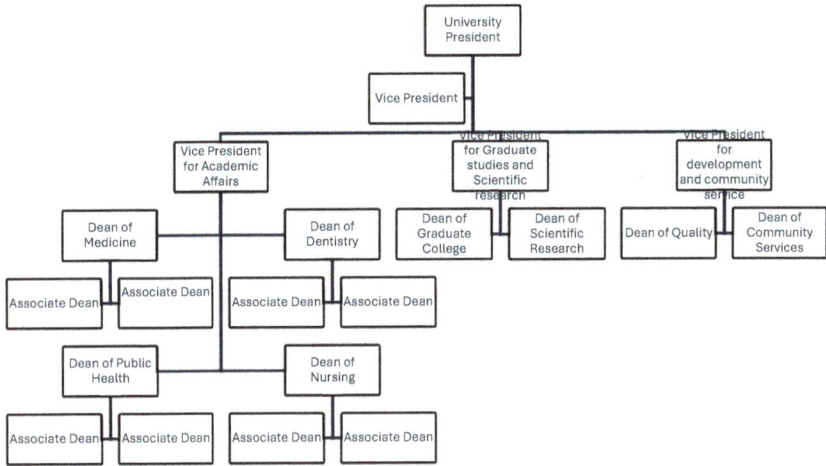

Figure 1.1: Vertical Organizational Chart

Horizontal Organizational Chart

A horizontal organizational chart, or flat organizational chart, features a less defined chain of command. In this structure, employees often report to multiple supervisors and share similar duties. This model promotes collaboration and flexibility, reducing the layers of management and encouraging a more egalitarian approach to decision-making (Forbes, 2024).

An example explained in figure 1.2 of a horizontal Organizational chart In this chart:

- The **CEO** is at the top and could hold several administrative roles.
- **Head of clinical Department:** report directly to the hospital's CEO are directly below the CEO without an intermediary administrative layer or level and oversee different clinical teams.
- Each **Team** works independently and could collaborate with other teams if necessary.

This structure helps improve communication, speeds up decision-making, and empowers employees to take more responsibility.

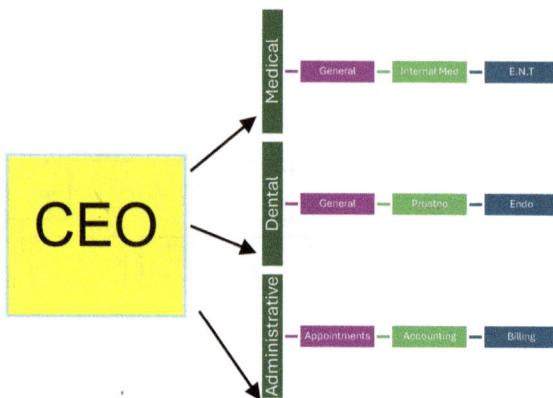

Figure 1.2: Horizontal organizational chart

Empowerment

Empowerment is also Known as the Delegation of Power. Empowerment in organizational contexts is often synonymous with the delegation of power. This concept involves transferring decision-making authority from higher levels of management to lower levels, including frontline employees. Empowerment aims to enhance employees' autonomy and responsibility, allowing them to make decisions that directly affect their work and the organization (Jong & Faerman, 2021).

Decisions Are Not Centralized

In an empowered organization, decisions are decentralized rather than centralized. This means that decision-making authority is distributed throughout the organization, rather than being concentrated at the top. Decentralization allows employees at various levels to participate in decision-making processes, which can lead to more responsive and adaptive organizational practices (Brinkerhoff & Azfar, 2006).

Less Bureaucracy

Empowerment reduces bureaucracy by minimizing the layers of management and the rigidity of hierarchical structures. This reduction in bureaucracy can lead to increased efficiency and faster decision-making, as employees are able to address issues and implement solutions without needing to navigate through multiple levels of approval (Brinkerhoff &

Azfar, 2006). Additionally, less bureaucracy can enhance employee motivation and job satisfaction, as they feel more valued and involved in the organization's success (Jong & Faerman, 2021).

References:

1. Academy of Nutrition and Dietetics. (2023). Nutrition Care Manual. Academy of Nutrition and Dietetics.
2. American Hospital Association. (2021). Fast Facts on U.S. Hospitals 2021. AHA.
3. American Hospital Association. (2024). Fast Facts on U.S. Hospitals 2024. AHA
4. American Society of Health-System Pharmacists. (2023). ASHP Guidelines on the Pharmacy and Therapeutics Committee and the Formulary System. ASHP.
5. Boardable. (2024). How Governing Boards Work in the Healthcare Industry. Retrieved from https://boardable.com/resources/governing-boards-in-healthcare/
6. Boardeffect. (2018). Roles & Responsibilities of a Board of Directors for a Hospital. Retrieved from https://www.boardeffect.com/blog/roles-responsibilities-board-directors-hospital/
7. Brinkerhoff, D. W., & Azfar, O. (2006). Decentralization and Community Empowerment: Does Community Empowerment Deepen Democracy and Improve Service Delivery? U.S. Agency for International Development.
8. Burke, L. G., Frakt, A. B., Khullar, D., Orav, E. J., & Jha, A. K. (2017). Association Between Teaching Status and Mortality in US Hospitals. JAMA.
9. Centers for Medicare & Medicaid Services. (2024). Hospitals. CMS.
10. Definitive Healthcare. (2024). How big is the average U.S. hospital? Definitive Healthcare.
11. Forrest, C. B. (2003). Primary Care Gatekeeping and Referrals: Effective Filter or Failed Experiment? BMJ.
12. Forbes. (2024). 7 Organizational Structure Types (With Examples). Retrieved from https://www.forbes.com/advisor/business/organizational-structure/
13. Gallagher Healthcare. (2018). What Are the Different Types of Hospitals? Gallagher Healthcare.
14. Garg, P. P., Frick, K. D., Diener-West, M., & Powe, N. R. (2014). Effect of the Ownership of Dialysis Facilities on Patients' Survival and Referral for Transplantation. New England Journal of Medicine.

15. Geriatric Academy. (2024). Acute Care Vs Long Term Care: What Is The Difference? Retrieved from https://geriatricacademy.com/long-term-care-and-acute-care-difference/

16. HealthIT.gov. (2023). Benefits of EHRs. HealthIT.gov.

17. HealthLeaders. (2019). 3 Strategic Differences Between Nonprofit and For-Profit Hospitals.

18. Healthline. (2023). Outpatient vs. Inpatient Surgery. Retrieved from https://www.healthline.com/health/outpatient-vs-inpatient-surgery

19. Healthcare Dive. (2017). Nonprofit For-Profit Hospitals Play Different Roles but See Similar Financial Outcomes.

20. Jong, J., & Faerman, S. R. (2021). Centralization and Decentralization: Balancing Organizational and Employee Expectations. In Global Encyclopedia of Public Administration, Public Policy, and Governance. Springer.

21. Liu, J. B., Kelz, R. R., & Kelz, M. S. (2018). Types of Hospitals in the United States. JAMA.

22. Medical News Today. (2024). Acute vs. chronic conditions: How are they different? Retrieved from https://www.medicalnewstoday.com/articles/acute-vs-chronic-conditions

23. Mount Sinai. (2014). How Different Are For-Profit and Nonprofit Hospitals?

24. National Council on Aging. (2024). Chronic vs. Acute Medical Conditions: What's the Difference? Retrieved from https://www.ncoa.org/article/chronic-versus-acute-disease/

25. Popowitz, E. (2023). The Difference Between Non-Profit and For-Profit Hospitals. Definitive Healthcare.

26. Saultz, J. W. (2000). Textbook of Family Medicine. McGraw-Hill.

27. Shi, L., & Singh, D. A. (2022). Essentials of the U.S. Health Care System. Jones & Bartlett Learning.

28. Starfield, B. (1998). Primary Care: Balancing Health Needs, Services, and Technology. Oxford University Press.

29. Texas Healthcare Trustees. (2017). Mergers and Affiliations 101: Why Hospitals Choose This Path and Key Considerations for Success.

30. The Joint Commission. (2024). Hospital Accreditation. The Joint Commission.

31. Torrey, T. (2024). Primary, Secondary, Tertiary, and Quaternary Care. Verywell Health.

32. Venngage. (2023). Organizational Chart: Types, Purpose & 20 Real-Life Examples. Retrieved from https://venngage.com/blog/organizational-chart-examples/

33. Welch, W. P., Xu, L., De Lew, N., & Sommers, B. D. (2023). Ownership of Hospitals: An Analysis of Newly-Released Federal Data & A Method for Assessing Common Owners. ASPE.

34. Zheng, K. (2023). For-Profit Hospitals vs. Nonprofit: Key Differences. IntelyCare.

Chapter 2

Leadership, Management, and Governance

The basic working structure in healthcare is often represented as a triangle, comprising three main entities: the Governing Body, Administration, and Medical Staff. This structure ensures that healthcare organizations operate efficiently and provide high-quality care.

Governing Body

The Governing Body, also known as the board of trustees, board of directors, board of governance, or governing board, is ultimately responsible for the quality of care provided by the healthcare organization (American College of Healthcare Executives, 2024). The Governing Body's primary role is to create and maintain an internal environment where all members can fully engage in achieving the organization's objectives (American College of Healthcare Executives, 2024). Managers and quality professionals are tasked with developing programs and systems to meet these objectives.

Functions of the Governing Body

The Governing Body functions as an active and effective board of directors, overseeing the hospital or health organization. It ensures that the organization provides quality care, for example, by overseeing credentialing processes (Functionly, 2024). Additionally, the Governing

Body is responsible for the financial well-being of the organization, with the Chief Quality Officer (CQO) reporting to the Governing Body via the Chief Executive Officer (CEO) (Functionly, 2024).

Corporate bylaws

Corporate bylaws are essential documents that outline the rules and regulations governing a corporation's operations. They provide a framework for how the organization works and operates, detailing its purpose, the duties and responsibilities of its employees, and the rights and responsibilities of shareholders. Additionally, bylaws specify the procedures for the removal of officers and directors and outline the authority and responsibility of each managerial level, particularly concerning quality management (Legal Templates, 2023).

How Organizations Work and Operate

Corporate bylaws define the internal management structure of a corporation, including the roles and responsibilities of the board of directors, officers, and employees. They establish procedures for meetings, voting, and decision-making processes, ensuring that the organization operates smoothly and efficiently (Rocket Lawyer, 2024).

Organizational Purpose

The bylaws articulate the corporation's purpose, which guides its strategic direction and operational goals. This purpose is often aligned with the corporation's mission and vision statements, providing a clear framework for decision-making and organizational activities (Rocket Lawyer, 2024).

Duties and Responsibilities

Bylaws specify the duties and responsibilities of the corporation's employees, officers, and directors. This includes outlining job descriptions, performance expectations, and reporting relationships. By clearly defining these roles, bylaws help ensure accountability and effective management within the organization (Wall Street Mojo, 2024).

Shareholders' Rights and Responsibilities

In corporations with shareholders, bylaws detail the ownership rights and responsibilities of these stakeholders. This includes information on voting rights, dividend distribution, and procedures for transferring shares. Bylaws also outline the processes for holding annual and special meetings of shareholders (Rocket Lawyer, 2024).

Removal of Officers and Directors

Corporate bylaws provide procedures for the removal of officers and directors, ensuring that there is a clear and fair process in place. This can include specifying the grounds for removal, the process for calling a meeting to vote on removal, and the required majority for such a vote (Legal Templates, 2023).

Quality Management and bylaws

Regarding quality management, bylaws specify the authority and responsibility of each managerial level. This ensures that quality standards are maintained throughout the organization and that there is a clear chain of command for addressing quality issues. By defining these roles, bylaws help promote a culture of continuous improvement and accountability (Wall Street Mojo, 2024).

Leadership versus Management

Leadership and management are often used interchangeably, but they encompass distinct roles and responsibilities, especially in the healthcare sector. While there is some overlap, the focus and functions of leaders and managers differ significantly.

Are Leaders and Managers the Same People?

Leaders and managers can be the same individuals, but their roles are distinct. Leaders are primarily focused on setting a vision, inspiring, and guiding others towards achieving long-term goals. They are often seen as change agents who look beyond the immediate tasks to the broader organizational objectives (Limb, 2016). Managers, on the other hand, are more concerned with the day-to-day operations, ensuring that the organizational processes run smoothly and efficiently (Stewart, 2023).

Healthcare's Special Need for Both

Healthcare organizations require both strong leadership and effective management to ensure high-quality patient care and operational efficiency. Leaders in healthcare are responsible for strategic planning, policy development, and fostering a culture of continuous improvement. They focus on external factors such as regulatory changes, technological advancements, and patient care trends (Baginski, 2023). Managers, however, handle the internal operations, including staffing, budgeting, and compliance with healthcare standards (Stewart, 2023).

Leader Focus is More External to the Organization

Leaders in healthcare often focus on external factors that influence the organization. They are involved in strategic initiatives, community engagement, and partnerships with other healthcare entities. Their role includes anticipating future challenges and opportunities, and aligning the organization's goals with these external factors (Limb, 2016). This external focus helps in navigating the complex healthcare environment and ensuring the organization remains competitive and innovative.

Crossover into Various Areas

There is a significant crossover between leadership and management roles in healthcare. Effective leaders need to understand management principles to implement their vision successfully. Similarly, managers often need leadership skills to motivate their teams and drive organizational change (Limb, 2016). This crossover ensures that healthcare organizations can adapt to changes and maintain high standards of care.

Differences Between Administrators, Leaders, and Managers

Administrators in healthcare are responsible for overseeing the entire operation of healthcare facilities. They ensure that the organization complies with laws and regulations, manages budgets, and oversees the implementation of policies. Leaders, as mentioned, focus on strategic vision and external relationships, while managers handle the operational aspects (Stewart, 2023).

Needs and Functions of Each in Healthcare Quality

- **Administrators:** Ensure compliance with healthcare regulations, manage financial resources, and oversee policy implementation. Their role is crucial in maintaining the legal and financial health of the organization.
- **Leaders:** Drive strategic initiatives, foster innovation, and build external relationships. They play a key role in setting the direction for the organization and ensuring it adapts to external changes.
- **Managers:** Handle day-to-day operations, manage staff, and ensure efficient use of resources. They are essential for maintaining the operational efficiency and quality of patient care.

Manager	Leader
Has subordinates	Has followers
Drive People	Inspire and influence People
Follows Policy	Visionary
Says "I"	Says " WE"
Says " GO"	Says " Lets Go"
Reactive	Proactive
Authority style	Charismatic style

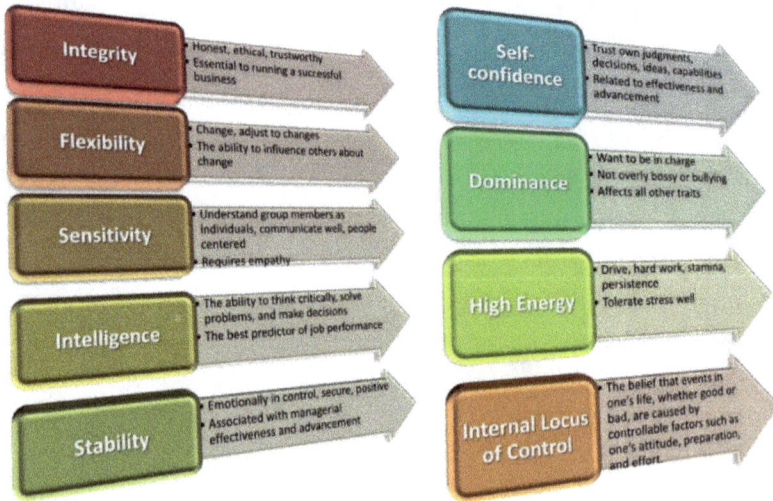

Integrity • Honest, ethical, trustworthy • Essential to running a successful business

Flexibility • Change, adjust to changes • The ability to influence others about change

Sensitivity • Understand group members as individuals, communicate well, people centered • Requires empathy

Intelligence • The ability to think critically, solve problems, and make decisions • The best predictor of job performance

Stability • Emotionally in control, secure, positive • Associated with managerial effectiveness and advancement

Self-confidence • Trust own judgments, decisions, ideas, capabilities • Related to effectiveness and advancement

Dominance • Want to be in charge • Not overly bossy or bullying • Affects all other traits

High Energy • Drive, hard work, stamina, persistence • Tolerate stress well

Internal Locus of Control • The belief that events in one's life, whether good or bad, are caused by controllable factors such as one's attitude, preparation, and effort.

Figure 2.1: Nine Traits of Effective Leaders

Leadership Competencies

Leadership competencies are essential for effective leadership, particularly in the healthcare sector. These competencies enable leaders to navigate complex environments, inspire their teams, and drive organizational success.

More Forward Thinking

Leaders are inherently forward-thinking, focusing on long-term goals and future opportunities. This competency involves anticipating changes in the healthcare landscape, such as technological advancements and regulatory shifts, and preparing the organization to adapt accordingly (American College of Healthcare Executives [ACHE], 2024).

Set Direction for the Organization

Setting a clear direction is a fundamental competency for leaders. This involves developing a strategic vision and aligning the organization's goals with this vision. Effective leaders communicate this direction clearly to ensure that all team members understand and are committed to the organization's objectives (ACHE, 2024).

Motivate Employees and Stakeholders

Motivating employees and stakeholders is crucial for achieving organizational goals. Leaders use various strategies to inspire and engage their teams, such as recognizing achievements, providing opportunities for professional growth, and fostering a positive work environment (Tanner, 2001). This competency is vital for maintaining high levels of morale and productivity.

Keep Entity on Course

Leaders must ensure that the organization stays on course towards its strategic goals. This involves monitoring progress, making necessary adjustments, and addressing any obstacles that may arise. Effective leaders are adept at problem-solving and decision-making, ensuring that the organization remains focused and resilient (ACHE, 2024).

Effective Spokesperson

Being an effective spokesperson is another key competency. Leaders represent the organization to external stakeholders, including the community, regulatory bodies, and other healthcare entities. They must communicate effectively, build relationships, and advocate for the organization's interests (ACHE, 2024).

Determine Strategies for Future

Leaders are responsible for determining strategies that will guide the organization into the future. This involves analyzing trends, assessing risks, and developing plans that leverage the organization's strengths and opportunities. Strategic thinking is essential for ensuring long-term success and sustainability (ACHE, 2024).

Transform Organization

Transformational leadership is about driving significant change within the organization. Leaders with this competency inspire innovation, encourage new ways of thinking, and lead initiatives that improve processes and outcomes. This ability to transform the organization is critical in the dynamic and ever-evolving healthcare sector (Tanner, 2001).

Leadership roles in healthcare organizations

Chief Executive Officer (CEO)

The Chief Executive Officer (CEO) in healthcare is the highest-ranking executive responsible for the overall management and strategic direction of the organization. The CEO oversees all operations, ensures compliance with healthcare regulations, and works closely with the board of directors to implement policies and strategies. Key responsibilities include financial management, human resources oversight, and maintaining high standards of patient care (BoardEffect, 2018). CEOs must also navigate complex regulatory environments and foster relationships with stakeholders to ensure the organization's success (USC EMHA Online, 2023).

Chief Operating Officer (COO)

The Chief Operating Officer (COO) in healthcare is responsible for the day-to-day operations of the organization. This role involves overseeing various departments, ensuring efficient workflow, and implementing operational strategies to improve patient care and organizational performance. The COO works closely with the CEO to develop and execute long-term strategic plans and is often involved in budgeting, staffing, and compliance with healthcare standards (IntelyCare, 2023). The COO also plays a crucial role in fostering collaboration among departments to enhance patient outcomes (Dimitroff, 2023).

Chief Quality Officer (CQO)

The Chief Quality Officer (CQO) focuses on maintaining and improving the quality of patient care within the healthcare organization. This role involves monitoring clinical performance, implementing quality improvement initiatives, and ensuring compliance with regulatory standards. The CQO works closely with other executives to develop strategies that enhance patient safety and care quality. Key responsibilities include data collection and analysis, performance improvement, and fostering a culture of continuous improvement (Wolters Kluwer, 2020). The CQO also plays a vital role in achieving high-quality outcomes necessary for reimbursement and patient satisfaction (IntelyCare, 2023).

Chief Financial Officer (CFO)

The Chief Financial Officer (CFO) in healthcare is responsible for managing the financial health of the organization. This includes overseeing budgeting, financial planning, and reporting, as well as ensuring compliance with financial regulations. The CFO works closely with other executives to develop strategies that support the organization's financial stability and growth. Key responsibilities include managing revenue cycles, investment planning, and financial risk management (Deloitte Insights, 2022). The CFO also plays a critical role in addressing macroeconomic challenges and ensuring the organization's financial sustainability (HFMA, 2019).

Chief Technology Officer (CTO)

The Chief Technology Officer (CTO) in healthcare is responsible for overseeing the organization's technology infrastructure and strategy. This role involves implementing and managing technology systems that support patient care, data management, and operational efficiency. The CTO works closely with other executives to integrate innovative technologies such as electronic health records (EHRs), telemedicine, and data analytics into the healthcare system. Key responsibilities include cybersecurity, data privacy, and ensuring compliance with technology-related regulations (DigitalDefynd, 2024). The CTO also leads efforts to enhance patient care through technological advancements (Clearstep, 2022).

Chief Medical Officer (CMO)

The Chief Medical Officer (CMO) oversees the clinical operations of the healthcare organization, ensuring the delivery of high-quality medical care. This role involves acting as a liaison between the medical staff and the administration, developing clinical policies, and overseeing medical staff performance. The CMO is responsible for ensuring that clinical practices comply with regulatory standards and that patient care is both effective and efficient. Key responsibilities include quality improvement, clinical governance, and fostering a culture of evidence-based practice (Sonnenberg, 2018). The CMO also plays a crucial role in aligning clinical operations with the organization's strategic goals (JAMA Health Forum, 2022).

Edward Deming's Leadership importance in Quality
a Story with an S&P 500 Company

W. Edwards Deming, a renowned statistician and quality management guru, is well-known for his contributions to the field of quality control and management. One notable story involves his interaction with an S&P 500 company, where he decided to leave after realizing that the leadership was not committed to his principles.

In the early 1980s, Deming was invited to work with a major American automotive manufacturer, which was part of the S&P 500. The company was struggling with quality issues and sought Deming's expertise to improve their processes. Deming agreed to help and began his work by conducting seminars and workshops to educate the company's executives and employees on his principles of quality management (Deming, 1986).

Deming's approach emphasized the importance of top management's commitment to quality. He believed that for any significant improvement to occur, the leadership had to be fully engaged and supportive of the changes. During his time with the company, Deming observed that the CEO and other top executives were not present at his seminars and showed little interest in his teachings. This lack of engagement from the leadership was a red flag for Deming.

Realizing that the necessary commitment from the top was absent, Deming decided to terminate his involvement with the company. He believed that without the active participation and support of the leadership, his efforts would be futile. Deming's departure underscored his principle that quality improvement must start at the top and that leaders must be fully invested in the process (Deming, 1986).

This story highlights Deming's unwavering commitment to his principles and his belief in the critical role of leadership in driving quality improvement. It also serves as a reminder to organizations that true transformation requires the dedication and involvement of their leaders.

Fellowship: Complementary to Leadership

Fellowship is an essential component of effective leadership. It emphasizes the interdependent relationship between leaders and followers, highlighting that leadership cannot exist without followership.

For Every Leader, Need a Follower

For leadership to be effective, there must be followers who support and implement the leader's vision. This relationship is symbiotic, where followers play a crucial role in the success of leadership initiatives. According to Kelley (1992), effective followers are active participants who contribute to the organization's goals with enthusiasm and intelligence.

Not Everyone Can or Should Be a Leader

Not everyone is suited to be a leader, and that is perfectly acceptable. The effectiveness of an organization depends on having a balance of leaders and followers. Some individuals excel in supportive roles, providing the necessary foundation for leaders to succeed. This diversity in roles ensures that all aspects of the organization are covered (Kelley, 1992).

True Leaders Inspire Commitment

True leaders have the ability to inspire commitment and dedication among their followers. They do this by creating a compelling vision and fostering a sense of purpose. This inspiration leads to higher levels of engagement and productivity within the organization (Kouzes & Posner, 2017). Leaders who inspire commitment are often seen as role models, and their followers are more likely to go above and beyond in their duties.

Leaders Can't Be Self-Absorbed

Effective leaders are not self-absorbed; they prioritize the needs and well-being of their followers. This approach is aligned with the principles of servant leadership, where the leader's primary goal is to serve others (Greenleaf, 2002). Leaders who focus on the development and success of their followers create a positive and productive organizational culture.

Recognize Importance of Getting Respect

Gaining respect is crucial for leaders to maintain their influence and effectiveness. Respect is earned through consistent actions that demonstrate integrity, competence, and concern for others. Leaders who are respected by their followers are more likely to achieve their organizational goals and foster a collaborative environment (Kouzes & Posner, 2017).

Leadership types and styles

Transactional Leadership

Transactional leadership is a style that is highly task and result-driven. Leaders using this approach focus on the performance of their employees, regularly evaluating their work and providing rewards or punishments based on their performance. This style is effective in environments where tasks are routine and require strict adherence to procedures (AdventHealth University, 2020). Transactional leaders set clear goals and expectations, and employees are motivated by the rewards they receive for meeting these goals (CUNE, 2022).

Transformational Leadership

Transformational leadership is characterized by leaders who inspire and enthuse their employees. These leaders lead by example, maintain high levels of communication, and motivate their workers through non-financial means. Transformational leaders focus on the growth and development of their team members, encouraging innovation and creativity (Gabel, 2013). This style is particularly effective in healthcare settings where continuous improvement and adaptation to change are crucial (ANA Enterprise, 2023).

Bureaucratic Leadership

Bureaucratic leadership is defined by a strict adherence to rules and procedures. Leaders who adopt this style expect their employees to follow established guidelines precisely, leaving little room for innovation. This style is commonly used in government and public sectors to ensure compliance and reduce corruption (AIHR, 2023). However, it can lead to frustration among self-motivated employees who may feel stifled by the lack of flexibility (Segel, 2017).

Autocratic Leadership

Autocratic leadership, also known as authoritarian leadership, involves leaders having full control over decision-making processes. This style is effective in situations that require quick decisions, such as in military operations or surgical settings (NursingProcess.org, 2023). However, it can negatively impact the morale of creative employees who may feel their input is undervalued (HealthStream, 2021).

Charismatic Leadership

Charismatic leadership relies on the leader's ability to inspire and motivate their team through their personality and communication skills. Charismatic leaders are often experienced in their field and use their expertise to guide and influence their team (Western Governors University, 2021). This style is effective in building strong personal bonds with employees and motivating them to achieve high performance (The Bailey Group, 2021).

Laissez-Faire Leadership

Laissez-faire leadership is a hands-off approach where leaders delegate decision-making to their team members. This style is effective in highly motivated and experienced groups where team members are capable of working independently (University of Tulsa, 2024). However, it can lead to issues if team members lack the necessary experience or motivation (Steinhauer, 2020).

Democratic/Participative Leadership

Democratic leadership involves the distribution of power among team members, with leaders actively seeking input and participation from their team. Unlike laissez-faire leadership, the final decision-making power rests with the leader (NursingProcess.org, 2023). This style promotes collaboration and inclusivity, leading to higher job satisfaction and team cohesion (SNHU, 2024).

References:

1. AdventHealth University. (2020). 5 types of leadership styles in healthcare. https://www.ahu.edu/blog/leadership-styles-in-healthcare

2. AIHR. (2023). What is bureaucratic leadership? Plus examples. https://www.aihr.com/hr-glossary/bureaucratic-leadership/

3. American College of Healthcare Executives. (2024). Foundations of well-managed healthcare organizations. https://www.ache.org/

4. American College of Healthcare Executives. (2024). Healthcare leadership competencies. https://www.ache.org/about-ache/resources-and-links/healthcare-leadership-competencies

5. American College of Healthcare Executives. (2024). Understanding healthcare organizational structures. https://www.functionly.com/orginometry/healthcare/organizational-chart

6. ANA Enterprise. (2023). What is transformational leadership in nursing? https://www.nursingworld.org/content-hub/resources/nursing-leadership/transformational-leadership-in-nursing/

7. Baginski, R. M. (2023). Healthcare management vs. leadership: What's the difference? Northeastern University.

8. BoardEffect. (2018). The role of the CEO for healthcare industries. https://www.boardeffect.com/blog/role-ceo-healthcare-industries/

9. CUNE. (2022). 11 leadership styles in healthcare. https://www.cune.edu/academics/resource-articles/leadership-styles-healthcare

10. Deloitte Insights. (2022). The health care CFO's expanded role. https://www2.deloitte.com/us/en/insights/industry/health-care/health-care-finance-leaders-expanded-role.html

11. Deming, W. E. (1986). Out of the crisis. MIT Press.

12. DigitalDefynd. (2024). Role of CTO in the healthcare sector. https://digitaldefynd.com/IQ/role-of-cto-in-the-healthcare-sector/

13. Dimitroff, W. (2023). What does a chief operating officer do in healthcare? https://www.chiefoperatingofficer.io/what-does-a-chief-operating-officer-do-in-healthcare

14. Gabel, S. (2013). Transformational leadership and healthcare. Medical Science Educator, 23(1), 55-60.

https://med.stanford.edu/content/dam/sm/CME/documents/Gabel2013_Article_TransformationalLeadershipAndH.pdf

15. Greenleaf, R. K. (2002). Servant leadership: A journey into the nature of legitimate power and greatness. Paulist Press.

16. HFMA. (2019). The healthcare CFO of the future: How finance leaders are adapting to relentless change. https://www.hfma.org/leadership/financial-leadership/the-healthcare-cfo-of-the-future/

17. IntelyCare. (2023). Healthcare chief operating officer job description. https://www.intelycare.com/facilities/resources/healthcare-chief-operating-officer-job-description-template/

18. JAMA Health Forum. (2022). The growing role of chief medical officers in major corporations. https://jamanetwork.com/journals/jama-health-forum/fullarticle/2794537

19. Kelley, R. E. (1992). The power of followership: How to create leaders people want to follow, and followers who lead themselves. Doubleday.

20. Kouzes, J. M., & Posner, B. Z. (2017). The leadership challenge: How to make extraordinary things happen in organizations (6th ed.). Jossey-Bass.

21. Legal Templates. (2023). Corporate bylaws template. https://legaltemplates.net/form/corporate-bylaws/

22. Limb, M. (2016). How does leadership differ from management in medicine? BMJ, 352, i631. https://doi.org/10.1136/bmj.i631

23. Rocket Lawyer. (2024). Corporate bylaws: Make, sign & download. https://www.rocketlawyer.com/business-and-contracts/starting-a-business/incorporation/document/corporate-bylaws

24. Segel, K. T. (2017). Bureaucracy is keeping health care from getting better. Harvard Business Review. https://hbr.org/2017/10/bureaucracy-is-keeping-health-care-from-getting-better

25. SNHU. (2024). 5 leadership styles in nursing. https://www.snhu.edu/about-us/newsroom/health/5-leadership-styles-in-nursing

26. Sonnenberg, M. (2018). Changing roles and skill sets for chief medical officers. https://www.physicianleaders.org/articles/changing-roles-skill-sets-chief-medical-officers

27. Steinhauer, R. (2020). Laissez-faire leadership: You'd have to be crazy to be this kind of leader. Nursing Centered. https://nursingcentered.sigmanursing.org/features/more-features/Vol42_4_laissez-faire-leadership-you-d-have-to-be-crazy-to-be-this-kind-of-leader

28. Stewart, S. (2023). Healthcare management vs. leadership: What's the difference? Northeastern University.

29. Tanner, C. (2001). Key healthcare leadership competencies: Perspectives from current leaders. https://www.oha.com/Bulletins/Paper%208%20-%20Key%20Healthcare%20Leadership%20Competencies.pdf

30. The Bailey Group. (2021). The main leadership styles in healthcare. https://thebaileygroup.com/the-different-leadership-styles-in-healthcare-and-how-they-can-affect-your-organization/

31. University of Tulsa. (2024). Leadership styles in nursing. https://online.utulsa.edu/blog/leadership-styles-in-nursing/

32. USC EMHA Online. (2023). Chief executive officer job description and salary. https://healthadministrationdegree.usc.edu/careers-in-executive-health-administration/resources/chief-executive-officer-job-description/

33. Wall Street Mojo. (2024). Corporate bylaws – What are they, explained, examples, template. https://www.wallstreetmojo.com/corporate-bylaws/

34. Western Governors University. (2021). What is charismatic leadership? https://www.wgu.edu/blog/charismatic-leadership2103.html

35. Wolters Kluwer. (2020). The role of chief quality officer. https://www.wolterskluwer.com/en/expert-insights/the-role-of-chief-quality-officer

Chapter 3

<u>Quality Concepts</u>

Definition and Perspectives

Quality can be broadly defined as the degree to which a set of inherent characteristics fulfills requirements (International Organization for Standardization [ISO], 2015). This definition emphasizes the importance of meeting predefined standards and expectations. However, the interpretation of quality can vary significantly depending on the context.

In the context of products and services, quality often refers to the degree of excellence and the ability to satisfy customer needs (Juran, 1988). For instance, in manufacturing, quality might be measured by the durability and reliability of a product. In healthcare, it could be assessed by patient outcomes and satisfaction.

Historical Perspectives

The concept of quality has evolved over time. Prophet Muhammad PBUH says: "Verily, GOD loves that when anyone of you does a job, she/he should perfect it.", which is even a higher state than quality, as he refers to excellence. Excellence became a concept in quality and all services organizations including healthcare are rewarded for excellence in their performance with the Deming, Malcolm Baldrige, and King Abdulaziz Quality Awards in Japan, the United States, and Saudi Arabia respectively.

In the early 20th century post World War II, quality control was primarily focused on inspection and defect detection. Pioneers like W. Edwards Deming and Joseph Juran introduced the principles of quality management, emphasizing continuous improvement and customer satisfaction (Deming, 1986; Juran, 1988).

Quality in Different Disciplines

1. Manufacturing and Engineering: In these fields, quality is often associated with the precision and reliability of products. Standards such as Six Sigma and Total Quality Management (TQM) are widely used to ensure high-quality outputs (Montgomery, 2009).
2. Healthcare: Quality in healthcare is measured by patient outcomes, safety, and satisfaction. The Institute of Medicine (IOM) defines healthcare quality as the degree to which health services for individuals and populations increase the likelihood of desired health outcomes (IOM, 2001).
3. Education: In education, quality is often linked to the effectiveness of teaching methods and the achievement of learning outcomes. Accreditation bodies set standards to ensure educational institutions meet certain quality benchmarks (Middle States Commission on Higher Education [MSCHE], 2020).

Understanding Quality

Customer-Focused Quality

Quality is fundamentally customer-focused, meaning that the primary objective is to meet and exceed the needs and expectations of the customer. This perspective is central to modern quality management principles. According to the International Organization for Standardization (ISO), customer focus is the first principle of quality management, emphasizing that organizations should understand current and future customer needs, meet customer requirements, and strive to exceed customer expectations (ISO, 2015). This approach ensures that the products or services provided are aligned with what customers value most, thereby enhancing customer satisfaction and loyalty (Olanab, 2024).

Incremental Improvement

Quality is also about incremental improvement, often referred to as continuous improvement. This concept is rooted in the idea that organizations should constantly seek ways to improve their processes, products, and services. The philosophy of continuous improvement is a core component of methodologies such as Total Quality Management (TQM) and Lean Manufacturing. These methodologies advocate for small, ongoing positive changes that can lead to significant improvements over time (Montgomery, 2009). This approach not only helps in maintaining high standards but also in adapting to changing customer needs and market conditions.

Doing the Right Thing the First Time

Another key aspect of quality is doing the right thing the first time and doing it better the next. This principle is closely related to the concept of "right-first-time" (RFT) and is a critical element in quality assurance and control. The goal is to minimize errors and defects in the production process, thereby reducing waste and increasing efficiency. This principle is emphasized in Six Sigma, a data-driven approach to improving quality by identifying and eliminating defects in processes (Pyzdek & Keller, 2014). By focusing on getting things right the first time, organizations can save time and resources, and by continuously improving, they can enhance their performance and customer satisfaction.

Stakeholders' different Perspectives on Health Care Quality

Health care quality is a multifaceted concept that varies significantly depending on the perspectives of different stakeholders. These stakeholders include patients, health care providers, insurers, and policymakers, each of whom has unique priorities and definitions of what constitutes quality care. Understanding these differing perspectives is crucial for developing comprehensive and effective health care quality improvement strategies.

Patients' Perspective

From the patients' viewpoint, health care quality is often associated with the outcomes of care, the accessibility of services, and the interpersonal aspects of care. Patients typically prioritize aspects such as effective communication, empathy, and respect from health care providers. They value timely access to care and the ability to participate in decision-making processes regarding their treatment (Epstein & Street, 2011). For patients, quality care means receiving treatments that lead to positive health outcomes and experiencing a health care environment that is supportive and responsive to their needs.

Health Care Providers' Perspective

Health care providers, including doctors, nurses, and other medical professionals, often define quality in terms of clinical outcomes and adherence to evidence-based practices. They focus on the technical aspects of care, such as the accuracy of diagnoses, the effectiveness of treatments, and the minimization of medical errors (Donabedian, 1988). Providers also emphasize the importance of continuous professional development and the use of advanced medical technologies to enhance care quality.

Insurers' Perspective

Insurers view health care quality through the lens of cost-effectiveness and efficiency. They are concerned with the financial sustainability of health care services and the optimization of resource use. Insurers prioritize measures that reduce unnecessary treatments and hospitalizations, promote preventive care, and ensure that care is delivered in the most cost-effective settings (Porter & Teisberg, 2006). For insurers, high-quality care is synonymous with achieving the best health outcomes at the lowest possible cost.

Policymakers' Perspective

Policymakers focus on the broader public health implications of health care quality. They are concerned with ensuring equitable access to health care services, improving population health outcomes, and maintaining regulatory standards. Policymakers emphasize the importance of health care quality metrics and standards to monitor and improve the performance of health care systems (Institute of Medicine [IOM], 2001).

Measurable Quality

Objective Definition of Quality

Measurable quality can be defined objectively as compliance with, or adherence to, established standards. These standards provide a clear framework for evaluating the performance, effectiveness, and overall quality of products, processes, services, or systems. The International Organization for Standardization (ISO) defines quality as the degree to which a set of inherent characteristics fulfills requirements (ISO, 2015). This definition underscores the importance of meeting predefined criteria to ensure consistency and reliability in quality management.

Clinical Standards

In the clinical context, standards often take the form of practice parameters or protocols. These standards are designed to establish acceptable expectations for patient and organizational outcomes. For example, clinical practice guidelines developed by professional organizations provide evidence-based recommendations for the diagnosis and treatment of specific conditions (Institute of Medicine [IOM], 2011). Adherence to these guidelines helps ensure that patients receive care that is consistent with the best available evidence, thereby improving health outcomes and reducing variability in clinical practice.

Guidelines for Excellence

Standards serve as guidelines for excellence by setting benchmarks for performance and quality. They provide a basis for continuous improvement and help organizations identify areas where they can enhance their processes and outcomes. For instance, the ISO 9001:2015 standard emphasizes the importance of a quality management system (QMS) that integrates continuous improvement and customer satisfaction into every aspect of an organization's operations (ISO, 2015). By adhering to these standards, organizations can achieve higher levels of efficiency, effectiveness, and customer satisfaction.

Appreciative Quality

Comprehension and Appraisal of Excellence

Appreciative quality involves the comprehension and appraisal of excellence beyond minimal standards and criteria. This concept goes beyond merely meeting established benchmarks; it seeks to recognize and value exceptional performance and outcomes. Appreciative quality requires a nuanced understanding of what constitutes excellence in a given context, often relying on the subjective judgments of those with significant experience and expertise (Brown, 2006).

Judgments of Skilled Practitioners

The assessment of appreciative quality necessitates the judgments of skilled, experienced practitioners and sensitive, caring persons. These individuals bring a depth of knowledge and a keen sense of what constitutes high-quality care or performance. Their evaluations are often based on a combination of technical proficiency, professional experience, and an empathetic understanding of the needs and expectations of those they serve (Brown, 2006). This approach ensures that quality assessments are not solely based on quantitative metrics but also consider qualitative aspects that contribute to overall excellence.

Peer Review Bodies

Peer review bodies play a crucial role in determining the quality or non-quality of specific patient-practitioner interactions. These bodies rely on the judgments of like professionals to evaluate the performance of their peers. This process involves a thorough review of clinical practices, patient outcomes, and adherence to professional standards. The peer review process is essential for maintaining high standards of care and fostering a culture of continuous improvement within the healthcare system (Quizlet, 2024). By leveraging the expertise and insights of experienced practitioners, peer review bodies can provide a more comprehensive and accurate assessment of quality.

Perceptive Quality

Degree of Excellence Perceived by Recipients

Perceptive quality refers to the degree of excellence as perceived and judged by the recipient or observer of care, rather than by the provider. This concept emphasizes the subjective experience of the patient or observer, focusing on how care is received and interpreted. According to Brown (2006), perceptive quality is crucial because it captures the patient's perspective, which can significantly influence their overall satisfaction and perception of care quality.

Based on Degree of Caring

Perceptive quality is generally based more on the degree of caring expressed by physicians, nurses, and other staff than on the physical environment and technical competence. This aspect highlights the importance of interpersonal interactions and the emotional support provided by healthcare professionals. Studies have shown that patients often rate their care higher when they feel that their providers are empathetic, attentive, and genuinely concerned about their well-being (Epstein & Street, 2011). This perception can be more influential than the technical aspects of care, such as the facilities or the medical procedures performed.

Quality History

Mid 19th Century in the UK: Public Health Awareness of Sanitary Problems

In the mid-19th century, the UK saw a significant rise in public health awareness, particularly concerning sanitary conditions. This period marked the beginning of efforts to address the unsanitary living conditions that were prevalent in urban areas due to rapid industrialization and urbanization (National Archives, 2024).

Dr. Edwin Chadwick's Public Health Report on Sanitary Conditions

Dr. Edwin Chadwick, a prominent social reformer, published his influential report on the sanitary conditions of the laboring population in 1842. This report highlighted the dire state of public health and the link between poor sanitary conditions and disease. Chadwick's recommendations included the provision of clean water, improved drainage systems, and the establishment of local health boards to oversee public health measures (Chadwick, 1842).

Florence Nightingale's Correlation Between Nursing Care and Lower Mortality

Florence Nightingale, known as the founder of modern nursing, made significant contributions to healthcare during the Crimean War. She demonstrated that improved sanitary conditions and nursing care could drastically reduce mortality rates among soldiers. Her work laid the foundation for modern nursing practices and emphasized the importance of hygiene in healthcare settings (Nightingale, 2020).

Early 20th Century: Dr. Emory Grove's Survey of Hospitals

In the early 20th century, Dr. Emory Grove conducted a survey of 200 hospitals in the UK to study mortality rates in postoperative situations. Although he faced challenges in comparing variations in mortality due to the lack of standardized data, his work underscored the need for a standardized classification of diseases to improve healthcare outcomes (Lin et al., 2016).

Flexner Report in 1910

The Flexner Report, published in 1910 by Abraham Flexner, critically assessed the state of medical education in the United States and Canada. The report highlighted numerous deficiencies in medical training and called for significant reforms, including higher admission standards, better facilities, and a focus on scientific research. This report led to the closure of many substandard medical schools and the establishment of a more rigorous medical education system (Flexner, 1910).

Deficiencies in Healthcare and Medical Education

The early 20th century also saw widespread recognition of deficiencies in healthcare and medical education. These deficiencies included inadequate training, lack of standardized curricula, and insufficient clinical practice opportunities. Efforts to address these issues were driven by reports like the Flexner Report and subsequent reforms in medical education (Buja, 2019).

World War I

World War I had a profound impact on healthcare quality, leading to advancements in medical technology and practices. The war necessitated rapid improvements in surgical techniques, infection control, and the development of new medical treatments. These advancements were later integrated into civilian healthcare, significantly improving medical care standards (Nodjimbadem, 2017).

World War II

World War II significantly influenced the evolution of quality management, particularly through the contributions of W. Edwards Deming. During the war, the need for high-quality military equipment led to the development and implementation of rigorous quality control processes. Deming, an American statistician, played a crucial role in this transformation by introducing statistical quality control methods to improve production processes (Deming, 1986).

Deming's work gained prominence post-WWII when he was invited to Japan to help rebuild its economy. His teachings on quality control and management were instrumental in Japan's economic recovery and industrial success. Deming emphasized the importance of understanding and reducing variation in production processes, which led to higher quality products and greater efficiency (Deming, 1986). His methods were quickly adopted by Japanese industries, leading to what is often referred to as the Japanese economic miracle (Britannica, 2023).

The impact of Deming's work in Japan was highlighted in the 1980 NBC documentary "If Japan Can, Why Can't We?" This program showcased how Japanese companies, by following Deming's principles, achieved remarkable improvements in quality and productivity. The documentary spurred interest in Deming's methods in the United States, leading to a quality revolution in American industries (NBC, 1980).

Shewhart Cycle

The Shewhart Cycle, also known as the Plan-Do-Check-Act (PDCA) cycle, was developed by Walter A. Shewhart and later popularized by W. Edwards Deming. This iterative process is used for continuous improvement in quality management. It involves planning a change, implementing the change, checking the results, and acting on what is learned to make further improvements (Deming, 1986).

Deming

W. Edwards Deming was a key figure in the development of quality management principles. His work emphasized the importance of statistical process control and continuous improvement. Deming's 14 Points for Management provided a framework for improving quality and productivity in organizations (Deming, 1986).

JCAHO 1952

The Joint Commission on Accreditation of Healthcare Organizations (JCAHO), established in 1951, plays a crucial role in setting standards for healthcare quality and safety. JCAHO evaluates and accredits healthcare organizations, ensuring they meet rigorous standards for patient care and organizational performance (Joint Commission, 2024).

QA, QI, QC, and TQM: Are They the same and used Interchangeably?

Quality Assurance (QA), Quality Improvement (QI), Quality Control (QC), and Total Quality Management (TQM) are terms often used in the context of quality management, but they are not interchangeable. Each term has a distinct meaning and role within the quality management framework.

Quality Assurance (QA)

Quality Assurance is the process of ensuring that products and services meet specified requirements and standards. It involves systematic activities and processes designed to provide confidence that quality requirements will be fulfilled (ISO, 2015). QA includes planning, designing for quality, setting and communicating standards, and identifying indicators for performance monitoring and compliance to standards (GIM, 2024).

Assurance Activities

- Rounds
- Tracers
- Checklists
- Assessments
- Plans
- Risk Plans
- Infection control
- Procedures
- Standardization

These activities help ensure that processes are followed correctly and consistently, thereby maintaining the quality of products and services (GIM, 2024).

Quality Control (QC)

Quality Control is the process of inspecting and testing products to ensure they meet the required standards. It focuses on identifying defects in the final products and correcting them. QC is a subset of QA and involves operational techniques and activities used to fulfill quality requirements (ASQ, 2024).

Control Activities

- Monitoring
- Data dwelling and mining
- Data management
- Measuring Key Performance Indicators (KPIs)

These activities are essential for comparing actual performance against expected performance and taking corrective actions when necessary (WallStreetMojo, 2024).

Quality Improvement (QI)

Quality Improvement is a structured approach to evaluating and improving processes and systems. It involves continuous efforts to enhance performance and outcomes. QI processes are data-driven and focus on making incremental improvements over time (Smartsheet, 2023).

Improvement Activities

- Organizing structured processes
- Defining improvement teams
- Implementing changes based on data analysis

QI complements both QA and QC by focusing on long-term improvements and efficiency (Smartsheet, 2023).

Total Quality Management (TQM)

Total Quality Management is a comprehensive management approach that integrates QA, QC, and QI. TQM involves all employees in continuous improvement efforts to enhance processes, products, services, and the organizational culture. It is customer-focused and aims for long-term success through customer satisfaction (ASQ, 2024).

Quality Gurus

Edward Deming: 14 Points

W. Edwards Deming's 14 Points for Management are foundational principles for transforming business effectiveness. These points were first introduced in his book *Out of the Crisis* (Deming, 1986). The 14 points include: creating constancy of purpose, adopting the new philosophy, ceasing dependence on inspection, ending the practice of awarding business on price alone, improving constantly and forever, instituting training, instituting leadership, driving out fear, breaking down barriers between departments, eliminating slogans and targets, eliminating numerical quotas, removing barriers to pride of workmanship, instituting a vigorous program of education and self-improvement, and putting everyone in the company to work on the transformation (Deming, 1986).

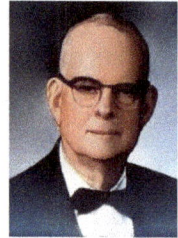

Joseph Juran: Trilogy

Joseph Juran's Quality Trilogy is a comprehensive framework for managing quality. The trilogy consists of three managerial processes: quality planning, quality control, and quality improvement (Juran, 1986). Quality planning involves identifying customers and their needs, developing product features that respond to those needs,

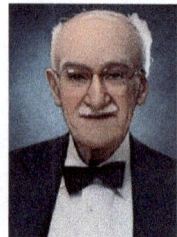

and designing processes capable of producing those features. Quality control focuses on monitoring operations to detect deviations from standards and taking corrective actions.

Quality improvement aims at achieving breakthrough improvements by identifying and addressing root causes of deficiencies (Juran, 1986).

Philip Crosby: 4 Absolutes (Zero Defects)

Philip Crosby's 4 Absolutes of Quality Management emphasize the **importance of conformance to requirements, prevention, zero defects, and measuring quality by the price of non-conformance** (Crosby, 1979). Crosby argued that quality should be defined as conformance to requirements, not as goodness. He believed that the system of quality is prevention, not appraisal. The performance standard must be zero defects, and the measurement of quality should be the price of non-conformance, not indices (Crosby, 1979).

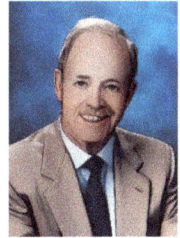

Walter Shewhart: GRANDFATHER & PDCA

Walter A. Shewhart is often referred to as the grandfather of statistical quality control. He developed the control chart and the concept of a state of statistical control (Shewhart, 1931). Shewhart also introduced the Plan-Do-Check-Act (PDCA) cycle, which was later popularized by W. Edwards Deming. The PDCA cycle is a continuous improvement process that involves planning, doing, checking, and acting to improve processes and products (Shewhart, 1939).

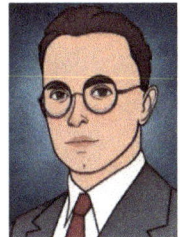

Florence Nightingale: Mother of Healthcare quality

Florence Nightingale is renowned for her contributions to modern nursing and healthcare reform. Her work during the Crimean War highlighted the importance of sanitation and hygiene in healthcare settings (Nightingale, 1859). Nightingale's efforts led to significant improvements in hospital conditions and patient care. She also established the Nightingale Training School for Nurses, which set the foundation for professional nursing education (Nightingale, 1860).

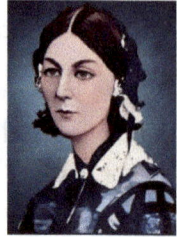

Avedis Donabedian: Father of Healthcare quality

Avedis Donabedian is best known for his work on quality in healthcare and the development of the Donabedian Model.

This model evaluates healthcare quality based on three components: structure, process, and outcomes (Donabedian, 1966). Structure refers to the attributes of the settings where care occurs, process denotes the methods of care delivery, and outcomes are the effects of healthcare on the health status of patients (Donabedian, 1966).

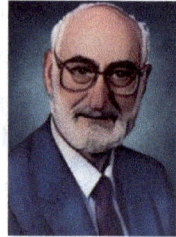

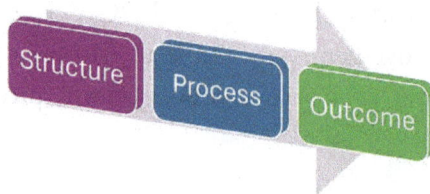

Figure3.1: The Donabedian Model

Donald Berwick: Healthcare and Patient Safety pioneer

Donald Berwick is a prominent figure in healthcare quality and patient safety. He co-founded the Institute for Healthcare Improvement (IHI) and has been a leading advocate for improving healthcare systems (Berwick, 2005). Berwick's work emphasizes the importance of patient-centered care, reducing medical errors, and implementing evidence-based practices to enhance patient safety and healthcare quality (Berwick, 2005).

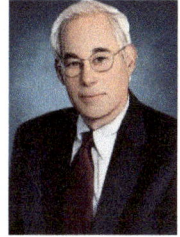

Quality in Healthcare

Healthcare Quality existed from mid 19th century by Florence Nightingale.

Florence Nightingale is widely recognized as a pioneer in healthcare quality. Her work during the Crimean War in the mid-19th century highlighted the importance of sanitation and hygiene in healthcare settings, leading to significant improvements in hospital conditions and patient care (Nightingale, 1859). She established the Nightingale Training School for Nurses, which laid the foundation for professional nursing education (Nightingale, 1860).

TQM in healthcare began in the US with Medicaid and Medicare in 1965.

Total Quality Management (TQM) in healthcare in the United States gained momentum with the introduction of Medicare and Medicaid in 1965. These programs, established under the Social Security Amendments of 1965, aimed to provide health insurance to the elderly and low-income individuals, respectively (National Archives, 1965). The implementation of these programs necessitated a focus on quality to ensure effective and efficient healthcare delivery.

During these times Joint Commission on Accreditation of Healthcare Organizations (JCAHO) was encouraged by the government to

enforce its accreditation requirements and tighten its standards for certifying the quality of hospitals.

The Joint Commission on Accreditation of Healthcare Organizations (JCAHO), now known as The Joint Commission, was encouraged by the government to enforce stricter accreditation requirements and standards for hospitals. This was part of the broader effort to improve healthcare quality following the establishment of Medicare and Medicaid (Joint Commission, 2023).

In 1966, Dr. Avedis Donabedian introduced his famous three measures of quality: Structure, process, and outcome.

Dr. Avedis Donabedian introduced a comprehensive model for evaluating healthcare quality in 1966, which includes three key components: structure, process, and outcome (Donabedian, 1966). He emphasized that healthcare organizations must consider all three measures when monitoring and assessing care quality.

Structure

Structure refers to the attributes of the settings where care occurs. Examples include:

- Number of board-certified physicians
- Patient-to-provider ratio
- Use of Electronic Medical Records (EMR)

Process

Process measures the methods of care delivery. Examples include:

- Percentage of patients who received immunizations
- Percentage of patients who received mammograms
- Percentage of diabetics who received blood tests

Outcome Measures

Outcome measures are the ultimate goals of healthcare and can be measured but only changed indirectly. Examples include:

- Number of wrong limbs amputated or wrong organs removed
- Percentage of patients who died from surgery
- Rate of surgical complications
- Rate of hospital-acquired infections (HAI)

References:

1. American Society for Quality (ASQ). (2024). Quality assurance vs quality control: Definitions & differences. Retrieved from https://asq.org/quality-resources/quality-assurance-vs-quality-control

2. Berwick, D. M. (2005). Improving patient care: The implementation of change in health care. BMJ Books.

3. Britannica. (2023). W. Edwards Deming. Retrieved from https://www.britannica.com/biography/W-Edwards-Deming

4. Brown, J. A. (2006). Healthcare quality concepts. DCA.

5. Buja, L. M. (2019). Medical education today: All that glitters is not gold. BMC Medical Education, 19(110). https://doi.org/10.1186/s12909-019-1535-9

6. Chadwick, E. (1842). Report on the sanitary conditions of the labouring population of Great Britain.

7. Crosby, P. B. (1979). Quality is free: The art of making quality certain. McGraw-Hill.

8. Deming, W. E. (1986). Out of the crisis. MIT Press.

9. Donabedian, A. (1966). Evaluating the quality of medical care. The Milbank Memorial Fund Quarterly, 44(3), 166-203.

10. Donabedian, A. (1988). The quality of care: How can it be assessed? Journal of the American Medical Association, 260(12), 1743-1748.

11. Epstein, R. M., & Street, R. L. (2011). The values and value of patient-centered care. Annals of Family Medicine, 9(2), 100-103.

12. Flexner, A. (1910). Medical education in the United States and Canada: A report to the Carnegie Foundation for the Advancement of Teaching. Carnegie Foundation.

13. Institute of Medicine (IOM). (2001). Crossing the quality chasm: A new health system for the 21st century. National Academies Press.

14. Institute of Medicine (IOM). (2011). Clinical practice guidelines we can trust. National Academies Press.

15. International Organization for Standardization (ISO). (2015). ISO 9001:2015 Quality management systems - Requirements. Retrieved from https://www.iso.org/standard/62085.html

16. Joint Commission. (2023). History of The Joint Commission. Retrieved from https://www.jointcommission.org/who-we-are/facts-about-the-joint-commission/history-of-the-joint-commission/

17. Juran, J. M. (1988). Juran on planning for quality. Free Press.

18. Lin, H. S., Watts, J. N., Peel, N. M., & Hubbard, R. E. (2016). Frailty and post-operative outcomes in older surgical patients: A systematic review. BMC Geriatrics, 16(157). https://doi.org/10.1186/s12877-016-0329-8

19. Middle States Commission on Higher Education (MSCHE). (2020). Standards for accreditation and requirements of affiliation. Retrieved from https://www.msche.org/standards/

20. Montgomery, D. C. (2009). Introduction to statistical quality control (6th ed.). Wiley.

21. National Archives. (1965). Medicare and Medicaid Act. Retrieved from https://www.archives.gov/milestone-documents/medicare-and-medicaid-act

22. National Archives. (2024). Public health and social policy in the 19th century. Retrieved from https://www.nationalarchives.gov.uk/help-with-your-research/research-guides/public-health-epidemics-19th-20th-centuries/

23. NBC. (1980). If Japan Can, Why Can't We? Retrieved from https://deming.org/if-japan-can-why-cant-we-1980-nbc-special-report/

24. Nightingale, F. (1859). Notes on hospitals. John W. Parker and Son.

25. Nightingale, F. (1860). Notes on nursing: What it is and what it is not. Harrison.

26. Nightingale, F. (2020). Florence Nightingale: Visionary for the role of clinical nurse specialist. OJIN: The Online Journal of Issues in Nursing, 25(2). https://doi.org/10.3912/OJIN.Vol25No02Man01

27. Nodjimbadem, K. (2017). How World War I influenced the evolution of modern medicine. Smithsonian Magazine. Retrieved from https://www.smithsonianmag.com/smithsonian-institution/how-world-war-i-impacted-modern-medicine-180962623/

28. Porter, M. E., & Teisberg, E. O. (2006). Redefining health care: Creating value-based competition on results. Harvard Business School Press.

29. Pyzdek, T., & Keller, P. A. (2014). The Six Sigma handbook (4th ed.). McGraw-Hill Education.

Chapter 4

Strategic Planning in Healthcare

A plan is defined as a predetermined course of action designed to achieve a prescribed goal or objective. Planning is a technical managerial function that enables organizations to deal with the present and anticipate the future. It involves developing a systematic approach for attaining the goals of the organization, which includes deciding what to do, as well as when, where, and how to do it (Robbins & Coulter, 2021).

Planning can be categorized into long-term and short-term planning. Long-term planning typically spans several years and is often the responsibility of senior management, while short-term planning focuses on immediate tasks and is handled by middle and first-line managers (Daft, 2020). It is every manager's duty to plan, and this function cannot be delegated to someone else (Jones & George, 2019).

Planning is considered a primary function and is the most critical management activity. Some managers are constantly confronting one crisis after another, likely because they did not plan or look ahead (Griffin, 2021). Effective planning helps managers anticipate future conditions, thereby reducing uncertainty and enabling them to think ahead about ways to overcome potential problems (Bateman & Snell, 2020).

Organization functions refer to all key governance, management, clinical, and support activities essential for the effective operation of an organization (Daft, 2020). Planning within these functions involves deciding in the present what actions to take to achieve desired outcomes in the future. This includes determining what to do, how to do it, when to do it, where to do it, and who will do it (Robbins & Coulter, 2021).

Planning is a continuous process that involves making choices about how to use available resources to achieve specific goals at some point in the future. This continuous nature of planning means that even after a plan is implemented, it should be revisited and adjusted based on new information and feedback, such as customer suggestions for new services (Jones & George, 2019). The initial phase of strategic planning involves setting goals and objectives, and analyzing events, trends, and customer needs. This phase is crucial as it lays the foundation for the entire planning process (Bateman & Snell, 2020).

The Importance of planning is multifaceted. It helps to anticipate the future, thus reducing uncertainty and enabling managers to think ahead about ways to overcome problems (Robbins & Coulter, 2021). Planning also helps define organizational goals and provides a framework to measure whether these goals have been achieved. This goal-setting process aligns the efforts of all members of the organization towards common objectives (Griffin, 2021). Additionally, planning aids in decision-making by helping managers choose from various alternatives, systematically analyzing options to make informed decisions that enhance organizational effectiveness (Daft, 2020). Efficient resource utilization is another critical aspect of planning, as it helps managers allocate resources in a way that maximizes their use and minimizes waste (Robbins & Coulter, 2021).

Elements of Planning

The Future

Planning inherently involves forecasting and preparing for future conditions. According to Koontz and O'Donnell (1976), planning is an intellectual process that involves the conscious determination of courses of action to achieve desired results. This process requires managers to anticipate future conditions and trends, which is supported by the work of

Fayol (1949), who emphasized that planning involves looking ahead and preparing for future contingencies.

Defined Goals

Setting clear and defined goals is a critical element of planning. Goals provide direction and a sense of purpose, guiding all subsequent planning activities. Drucker (1954) highlighted that effective planning begins with the establishment of clear objectives, which serve as benchmarks for measuring progress and success. Objectives must be specific, measurable, achievable, relevant, and time-bound (SMART) to be effective (Locke & Latham, 2002).

Making Choices

Planning involves making informed choices among various alternatives. This decision-making process is crucial for selecting the most appropriate course of action. Simon (1960) described decision-making as the heart of planning, where managers evaluate different options based on their potential outcomes and feasibility. The selection of the best alternative is essential for achieving the defined goals efficiently.

Efficient Use of Available Resources

Efficient resource utilization is a fundamental aspect of planning. Resources, including time, money, and human capital, must be allocated optimally to achieve the desired objectives. According to Robbins and Coulter (2012), planning helps in identifying the necessary resources and ensuring their efficient use, thereby minimizing waste and maximizing productivity. This aspect of planning is closely related to the concept of resource management, which involves the strategic allocation and utilization of resources to achieve organizational goals (Barney, 1991).

Continuous Review of Plans

Planning is not a one-time activity but a continuous process that requires regular review and adjustment. Mintzberg (1994) argued that plans must be flexible and adaptable to changing circumstances. Continuous review allows managers to assess the effectiveness of their plans and make necessary adjustments to stay on track. This iterative process ensures that plans remain relevant and aligned with the organization's goals and external environment.

Planning Classification

According to Time

Planning can be classified based on the time horizon into long-term, medium-term, and short-term plans. Long-term planning, which spans more than three years, involves setting strategic goals and objectives that guide the overall direction of an organization. This type of planning is crucial for addressing future uncertainties and ensuring sustainable growth (Mintzberg, 1994). Medium-term planning, covering one to three years, focuses on tactical goals that bridge the gap between strategic plans and day-to-day operations (Bryson, 2018). Short-term planning, which is less than one year, deals with operational goals and immediate tasks that need to be accomplished to support medium and long-term plans (Robbins & Coulter, 2012).

According to Organizational Level

Plans can also be classified based on the organizational level at which they are implemented. National plans are developed at the highest level and typically involve policies and strategies that affect the entire country. Regional plans are more localized and address the specific needs and conditions of a particular region (Friedmann, 2005). District plans are even more localized, focusing on smaller administrative units within a region. Hospital-wide plans encompass strategies and policies that affect the entire hospital, while departmental plans are specific to individual departments within the hospital (Hulshof et al., 2012).

According to Functional Area

Planning can be categorized based on the functional area it addresses. For instance, diagnostic service planning involves strategies to improve diagnostic capabilities and efficiency within a healthcare setting. Quality of care planning focuses on enhancing patient outcomes and ensuring high standards of care (Donabedian, 1988). Hospital information planning deals with the management and utilization of information systems to support hospital operations. Nursing planning involves strategies to optimize nursing staff allocation, training, and patient care (Aiken et al., 2002).

Planning Cycle

Planning

The planning phase involves setting objectives and determining the best course of action to achieve these goals. This phase is critical as it lays the foundation for all subsequent activities. According to Bryson (2018), effective planning requires a clear understanding of the organization's mission, vision, and strategic goals. This phase often involves environmental scanning, SWOT analysis (Strengths, Weaknesses, Opportunities, Threats), and the formulation of strategic plans (Mintzberg, 1994).

Implementation

Implementation is the process of putting the plan into action. This phase involves allocating resources, assigning tasks, and ensuring that all team members understand their roles and responsibilities. According to Kotter (1996), successful implementation requires effective communication, leadership, and the ability to manage change. It is during this phase that the theoretical aspects of the plan are translated into practical actions.

Evaluation

Evaluation involves assessing the effectiveness of the implemented plan. This phase is crucial for determining whether the objectives are being met and identifying any areas that need improvement. According to Patton (2008), evaluation should be systematic and based on predefined criteria and performance indicators. This phase often involves collecting and analyzing data to measure progress and outcomes.

Re-Planning

Re-planning, or the iterative process of revising plans, is essential for continuous improvement. This phase involves reviewing the results of the evaluation and making necessary adjustments to the plan. According to Mintzberg (1994), re-planning ensures that the organization remains adaptable and responsive to changing circumstances. This iterative process helps in refining strategies and improving overall effectiveness.

Why is Planning Avoided?

Laziness

Laziness, or a lack of motivation to engage in the planning process, can be a significant barrier. According to Steel (2007), procrastination, often linked to laziness, is a common reason why individuals avoid planning. Procrastinators tend to delay tasks that require effort and prefer immediate gratification over long-term benefits, which planning typically involves.

Lack of Commitment

A lack of commitment to the planning process can stem from various factors, including a lack of belief in the plan's effectiveness or a lack of personal investment in the outcomes. Meyer and Allen (1991) describe organizational commitment as a psychological state that characterizes an employee's relationship with their organization, which can influence their willingness to engage in planning activities. Without a strong commitment, individuals may not see the value in dedicating time and effort to planning.

Resistance to Change

Resistance to change is a well-documented phenomenon that can hinder planning efforts. Kotter (1996) explains that individuals often resist change due to fear of the unknown, loss of control, or disruption of routines. Planning often involves anticipating and preparing for change, which can be uncomfortable for those who prefer stability and predictability.

Fear of Failure

Fear of failure can be a powerful deterrent to planning. When individuals are afraid that their plans might not succeed, they may avoid planning altogether to protect themselves from potential disappointment and criticism. According to Conroy, Willow, and Metzler (2002), fear of failure is associated with anxiety and avoidance behaviors, which can prevent individuals from engaging in proactive planning.

Lack of Knowledge & Experience

A lack of knowledge and experience can make planning seem daunting and unmanageable. Individuals who are not familiar with the planning process or who lack the necessary skills may feel overwhelmed and unsure of where to start. According to Bandura (1997), self-efficacy, or the belief in one's ability to succeed, plays a crucial role in whether individuals engage in planning. Those with low self-efficacy may avoid planning due to a lack of confidence in their abilities.

Types of Plans

Strategic Plan

Strategic plans are long-range plans that typically cover a period of more than three years. They are broad in scope and are developed at the top levels of an organization. These plans are designed to align with the organization's mission and goals, providing a framework for long-term decision-making and resource allocation. According to Bryson (2018), strategic planning involves an analysis of the internal and external environments to identify opportunities and threats. This environmental analysis is crucial for setting realistic and achievable long-term objectives. Strategic plans often require marketing strategies to ensure that the organization can effectively reach its target audience and achieve its goals (Kotler & Keller, 2016).

Tactical Plan

Tactical plans are intermediate-range plans that typically cover a period of one to three years. These plans have a narrower scope compared to strategic plans and are more detailed. Tactical plans are developed at the middle management level and are designed to implement specific parts of the strategic plan. According to Robbins and Coulter (2012), tactical planning involves translating broad strategic goals into specific actions and short-term objectives. This type of planning ensures that the organization's strategic initiatives are effectively executed and that resources are allocated efficiently to achieve these goals.

Operational Plan

Operational plans are short-range plans that typically cover a period of less than one year. These plans have a very narrow scope and are focused on specific activities and tasks. Operational plans are developed at the lower management level and are concerned with the day-to-day operations of the organization. The primary concern of operational planning is efficiency rather than effectiveness, as it focuses on optimizing processes and ensuring that tasks are completed on time and within budget (Daft, 2016). According to Hill and Jones (2013), operational plans include detailed procedures and schedules that guide the daily activities of employees and ensure that the organization's short-term objectives are met.

Dependency of Planning Types

Strategic Planning

Strategic planning serves as the foundation for both tactical and operational planning. It involves setting long-term goals and determining the overall direction of the organization. According to Bryson (2018), strategic planning is essential for aligning the organization's mission and vision with its long-term objectives. This type of planning typically includes an environmental analysis to identify external opportunities and threats, which helps in formulating strategies that guide the organization towards its goals (Mintzberg, 1994).

Tactical Planning

Tactical plans are derived from strategic plans and focus on intermediate-range goals, usually spanning one to three years. These plans are more detailed and are developed at the middle management level. Tactical planning translates the broad objectives of strategic plans into specific actions and short-term objectives. According to Robbins and Coulter (2012), tactical plans are crucial for implementing the strategies outlined in the strategic plan and ensuring that resources are allocated efficiently to achieve these goals.

Operational Planning

Operational plans are based on tactical plans and focus on short-term objectives, typically covering less than one year. These plans are very specific and are developed at the lower management level. Operational planning involves detailed procedures and schedules that guide the day-to-day activities of the organization. The primary concern of operational planning is efficiency, as it aims to optimize processes and ensure that tasks are completed on time and within budget (Daft, 2016). Hill and Jones (2013) emphasize that operational plans are essential for achieving the short-term objectives that support the broader goals of tactical and strategic plans.

Proactive vs. Reactive Planning

Proactive Planning

Proactive planning is systematic, formalized, and anticipatory. It involves anticipating potential problems and opportunities and developing strategies to address them before they arise. According to Kotter (1996), proactive planning is essential for organizations to stay ahead of changes in the external environment and to capitalize on emerging opportunities. This type of planning requires a thorough analysis of internal and external factors and the development of contingency plans to mitigate risks (Bryson, 2018).

Reactive Planning

Reactive planning, on the other hand, is non-systematic and involves responding to events as they occur. This type of planning is not anticipatory and often involves making decisions under pressure. Reactive planning can be effective in addressing immediate issues, but it may lead to short-term fixes rather than long-term solutions. According to Mintzberg (1994), reactive planning can result in a more chaotic and less efficient response to problems, as it lacks the foresight and preparation that proactive planning provides.

Mission, Vision, and Values in Healthcare Organizations

Mission

A mission statement defines the core purpose and focus of an organization, describing what it does and for whom. It is a concise declaration of the organization's reason for existence. In healthcare, mission statements often emphasize patient care, community service, and the provision of high-quality medical services. For example, the mission of the Mayo Clinic is "to inspire hope and contribute to health and well-being by providing the best care to every patient through integrated clinical practice, education, and research" (Mayo Clinic, 2024). This statement highlights the organization's commitment to patient care and its integrated approach to healthcare delivery.

Vision

A vision statement outlines the desired future state of an organization. It is aspirational and forward-looking, providing a picture of what the organization aims to achieve in the long term. Vision statements in healthcare often focus on becoming leaders in medical innovation, improving patient outcomes, and expanding access to care. For instance, the vision of the Cleveland Clinic is "to be the world's leader in patient experience, clinical outcomes, research, and education" (Cleveland

Clinic, 2024). This vision statement sets a high standard for the organization and guides its strategic planning efforts.

Values

Values statements articulate the core principles and ethical standards that guide an organization's behavior and decision-making. In healthcare, values often include compassion, integrity, excellence, and respect for patients and staff. These values help create a positive organizational culture and ensure that all actions align with the organization's mission and vision. For example, the values of Johns Hopkins Medicine include "excellence and discovery, leadership and integrity, diversity and inclusion, and respect and collegiality" (Johns Hopkins Medicine, 2024). These values emphasize the importance of ethical conduct and continuous improvement in healthcare delivery.

Uses and Examples in Healthcare Organizations

Mission, vision, and values statements are essential tools for healthcare organizations. They provide a framework for strategic planning, guide decision-making, and help communicate the organization's goals and priorities to stakeholders. These statements also play a crucial role in shaping organizational culture and ensuring that all employees work towards common objectives.

For example, the mission statement of the Massachusetts General Hospital's Department of Neurology is "to provide outstanding clinical care while rapidly discovering new treatments to reduce and eliminate the devastating impact of neurological disorders" (Massachusetts General Hospital, 2024). This mission guides the department's clinical and research activities, ensuring that all efforts are aligned with the goal of improving patient outcomes.

Similarly, the vision statement of the University of New Mexico Hospital (UNMH) is "to be one of the nation's leading university hospitals that captures the synergy in being both an excellent academic institution and an innovative, community-oriented public teaching hospital" (University of New Mexico Hospital, 2024). This vision statement sets a high standard for the hospital and drives its efforts to achieve excellence in both education and patient care.

Values statements also play a critical role in healthcare organizations. For instance, the values of Seattle Children's Hospital include "collaboration, innovation, and respect" (Seattle Children's Hospital, 2024). These values guide the hospital's interactions with patients, families, and staff, fostering a culture of teamwork and continuous improvement.

SWOT Analysis

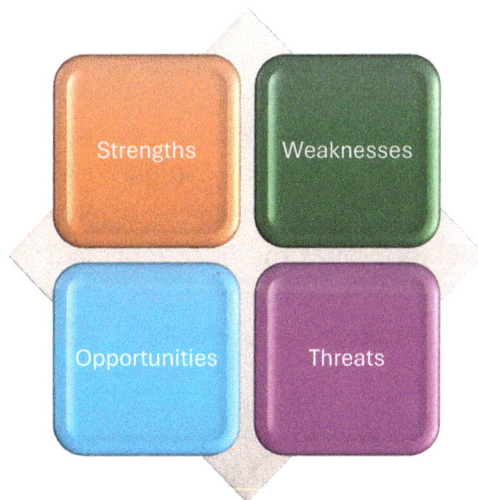

Figure 4.1 : SWOT Analysis

Internal Strengths

Strengths are internal attributes that give an organization a competitive advantage. These can include a strong brand reputation, skilled workforce, advanced technology, and robust financial resources. For example, a healthcare organization might have a highly qualified medical staff, state-of-the-art medical equipment, and a strong reputation for patient care (Barney, 1991). These strengths enable the organization to deliver high-quality services and maintain a competitive edge in the healthcare industry.

Internal Weaknesses

Weaknesses are internal factors that place an organization at a disadvantage relative to competitors. These can include outdated technology, high employee turnover, limited financial resources, and poor organizational structure. For instance, a hospital might struggle with inefficient administrative processes, leading to longer patient wait times and decreased patient satisfaction (Robbins & Coulter, 2012). Identifying weaknesses is crucial for developing strategies to mitigate these issues and improve overall performance.

External Opportunities

Opportunities are external factors that an organization can exploit to its advantage. These can include market growth, technological advancements, favorable regulatory changes, and partnerships. For example, a healthcare organization might benefit from advancements in telemedicine technology, allowing it to expand its services and reach more patients (Porter, 1985). Recognizing and capitalizing on opportunities can help an organization grow and enhance its competitive position.

External Threats

Threats are external factors that could harm an organization's performance. These can include economic downturns, increased competition, regulatory changes, and technological disruptions. For instance, changes in healthcare regulations or the emergence of new competitors can pose significant challenges to a hospital's operations (Kotler & Keller, 2016). Identifying threats allows an organization to develop contingency plans and strategies to mitigate potential risks.

Developing Goals and Objectives from SWOT Analysis

A SWOT analysis helps organizations develop their goals and objectives by providing a comprehensive understanding of their internal and external environments. By leveraging strengths, addressing weaknesses, capitalizing on opportunities, and mitigating threats, organizations can formulate strategic goals that align with their mission and vision (Bryson, 2018). For example, a hospital might set a goal to improve patient satisfaction by upgrading its technology and streamlining administrative processes, based on the insights gained from its SWOT analysis.

Governing Body

The governing body of a healthcare organization, also known as the board of trustees, board of directors, board of governance, or governing board, holds the ultimate responsibility for the quality of care provided. This body is tasked with creating and maintaining an internal environment that enables all members of the organization to be fully involved in achieving its objectives (Malik & Elorrio, 2023). Leaders within the organization must foster a culture that supports these goals, while managers and quality professionals develop the necessary programs and systems to achieve them (Robbins & Coulter, 2012).

Governing Body Quality Functions

The American Hospital Association (AHA) in 1982 outlined six broad categories of responsibilities and functions for the board:

1. **Organization**: Ensuring the organizational structure supports the mission and goals.
2. **Public Policy and External Relationships**: Engaging with external stakeholders and influencing public policy.
3. **Strategic Planning**: Setting long-term goals and strategies.
4. **Resource Management:** Overseeing the allocation and use of resources.
5. **Human Resource Development**: Ensuring the development and well-being of staff.
6. **Education and Research**: Promoting continuous learning and innovation (American Hospital Association, 1982).

Other Functions of the Governing Body

The governing body also has several other critical functions, including:

- Approving the organization's mission and vision.
- Approving the quality plan.
- Approving the organization's budget.
- Appointing senior personnel.
- Overseeing external contracts.
- Approving organizational policies.
- Being overall responsible for the organization's performance.
- Monitoring key programs such as safety and infection control (Malik & Elorrio, 2023).

Quality Council

The quality council in a healthcare organization is responsible for overseeing quality improvement efforts. This council maintains organizational focus on identified goals, fosters teamwork, and helps reduce internal competition. It also provides the necessary resources (human, equipment, financial) to achieve the quality vision and defines and publishes the council's responsibilities. Additionally, the council formulates quality improvement policies regarding quality priorities, participation, annual self-assessment, and reward and recognition systems (ASTHO, 2023).

Responsibilities of the Quality Council

- Providing official authority to quality improvement efforts.
- Maintaining organizational focus on identified goals.
- Fostering teamwork and reducing internal competition.
- Providing necessary resources to achieve the quality vision.
- Defining and publishing council responsibilities.
- Formulating quality improvement policies (ASTHO, 2023).

References:

1. Aiken, L. H., Clarke, S. P., Sloane, D. M., Sochalski, J., & Silber, J. H. (2002). Hospital nurse staffing and patient mortality, nurse burnout, and job dissatisfaction. JAMA, 288(16), 1987-1993.
2. American Hospital Association. (1982). Responsibilities of the Governing Body. Retrieved from https://www.aha.org
3. ASTHO. (2023). General Guidance to Support a Quality Improvement Council. Retrieved from https://www.astho.org/globalassets/pdf/general-guidance-to-support-a-quality-improvement-council.pdf
4. Bandura, A. (1997). Self-efficacy: The exercise of control. W.H. Freeman.
5. Barney, J. B. (1991). Firm resources and sustained competitive advantage. Journal of Management, 17(1), 99-120.
6. Bateman, T. S., & Snell, S. A. (2020). Management: Leading & Collaborating in a Competitive World. McGraw-Hill Education.
7. Bryson, J. M. (2018). Strategic Planning for Public and Nonprofit Organizations: A Guide to Strengthening and Sustaining Organizational Achievement. John Wiley & Sons.
8. Cleveland Clinic. (2024). Vision and Values. Retrieved from https://my.clevelandclinic.org/about/overview/mission-vision-values
9. Conroy, D. E., Willow, J. P., & Metzler, J. N. (2002). Multidimensional fear of failure measurement: The performance failure appraisal inventory. Journal of Applied Sport Psychology, 14(2), 76-90.
10. Daft, R. L. (2016). Management (12th ed.). Cengage Learning.
11. Daft, R. L. (2020). Management. Cengage Learning.
12. Donabedian, A. (1988). The quality of care: How can it be assessed? JAMA, 260(12), 1743-1748.
13. Drucker, P. F. (1954). The Practice of Management. Harper & Row.
14. Fayol, H. (1949). General and Industrial Management. Pitman Publishing.
15. Friedmann, J. (2005). Planning in the Public Domain: From Knowledge to Action. Princeton University Press.
16. Griffin, R. W. (2021). Management. Cengage Learning.
17. Hill, C. W. L., & Jones, G. R. (2013). Strategic Management: An Integrated Approach (11th ed.). Cengage Learning.
18. Hulshof, P. J. H., Kortbeek, N., Boucherie, R. J., Hans, E. W., & Bakker, P. J. M. (2012). Taxonomic classification of planning decisions in health care:

a structured review of the state of the art in OR/MS. Health Systems, 1(2), 129-175.

19. Johns Hopkins Medicine. (2024). Core Values. Retrieved from https://www.hopkinsmedicine.org/about/mission.html

20. Jones, G. R., & George, J. M. (2019). Essentials of Contemporary Management. McGraw-Hill Education.

21. Koontz, H., & O'Donnell, C. (1976). Management: A Systems and Contingency Analysis of Managerial Functions. McGraw-Hill.

22. Kotler, P., & Keller, K. L. (2016). Marketing Management (15th ed.). Pearson. Retrieved from https://www.pearson.com/store/p/marketing-management/P100000657568

23. Kotter, J. P. (1996). Leading Change. Harvard Business Review Press.

24. Locke, E. A., & Latham, G. P. (2002). Building a practically useful theory of goal setting and task motivation: A 35-year odyssey. American Psychologist, 57(9), 705-717.

25. Malik, A. M., & Elorrio, E. G. (2023). Governance and management in healthcare organizations: their different roles in driving safety and quality. International Journal for Quality in Health Care, 35(3), mzad046. https://doi.org/10.1093/intqhc/mzad046

26. Massachusetts General Hospital. (2024). Department of Neurology Mission Statement. Retrieved from https://www.massgeneral.org/neurology/about/mission

27. Mayo Clinic. (2024). Mission and Values. Retrieved from https://www.mayoclinic.org/about-mayo-clinic/mission-values

28. Meyer, J. P., & Allen, N. J. (1991). A three-component conceptualization of organizational commitment. Human Resource Management Review, 1(1), 61-89.

29. Mintzberg, H. (1994). The Rise and Fall of Strategic Planning. Free Press.

30. Patton, M. Q. (2008). Utilization-Focused Evaluation (4th ed.). SAGE Publications.

31. Porter, M. E. (1985). Competitive Advantage: Creating and Sustaining Superior Performance. Free Press. Retrieved from https://www.hbs.edu/faculty/Pages/item.aspx?num=193

32. Robbins, S. P., & Coulter, M. (2012). Management (11th ed.). Pearson. Retrieved from https://www.pearson.com/store/p/management/P100000657569

33. Robbins, S. P., & Coulter, M. (2021). Management. Pearson.

34. Seattle Children's Hospital. (2024). Our Values. Retrieved from https://www.seattlechildrens.org/about/mission-values/

35. Simon, H. A. (1960). The New Science of Management Decision. Harper & Brothers.

36. Steel, P. (2007). The nature of procrastination: A meta-analytic and theoretical review of quintessential self-regulatory failure. Psychological Bulletin, 133(1), 65-94.

37. University of New Mexico Hospital. (2024). Vision Statement. Retrieved from https://unmhealth.org/about/mission-vision-values.html

Chapter 5

Understanding Healthcare Directives

In healthcare there are many directives used for clinical and administrative purposes. In this chapter we shall understand the significance and use of all directives used in the medical context.

Policy

Policies serve as guiding principles that shape the provision of services and decision-making processes within organizations. They do not provide detailed instructions but rather set the framework within which decisions are made and actions are taken (de Leeuw, Clavier, & Breton, 2014). Policies are essential in healthcare settings as they ensure consistency, safety, and quality in service delivery (Unger, Morales, & De Paepe, 2020).

Administrative Policies in Healthcare

Administrative policies in healthcare address various operational aspects, such as staff utilization and organizational settings. For instance, policies may define who is qualified to perform specific medical procedures, such as cesarean sections. This involves establishing the scope of practice and determining the necessary qualifications for healthcare providers (Health Research Policy and Systems, 2014). Additionally, policies specify where procedures can be performed, ensuring that they are conducted in appropriate settings equipped with the necessary resources (BMC Health Services Research, 2020).

Health Care Services and Patient Safety

Policies also determine the availability of healthcare services and ensure patient safety. Decisions regarding the availability of services, such as cesarean sections, depend on the facility's capacity to manage high-risk cases, including the availability of trained personnel and equipment (Health Research Policy and Systems, 2014). Furthermore, policies outline procedures for maintaining patient safety during transfers between facilities, ensuring that patients receive continuous and safe care (BMC Health Services Research, 2020).

Examples of Healthcare Policies

1. **Cesarean Sections**: Policies may state that cesarean sections can be performed by credentialed physicians, including both general surgeons and obstetricians. These policies ensure that operating rooms are designated and equipped for such procedures, and that patients requiring intensive care are promptly referred to specialized facilities (Health Research Policy and Systems, 2014).
2. **Handwashing**: Effective handwashing is crucial for patient care. Policies ensure that handwashing facilities are available in patient care areas and that specific handwashing routines are followed to prevent infections (BMC Health Services Research, 2020).
3. **Visitor Policies**: To promote patient comfort and well-being, policies may limit the number of visitors and set age restrictions. These policies help maintain a conducive environment for patient recovery (Health Research Policy and Systems, 2014).
4. **Use of Transport Stretchers and Wheelchairs**: Policies ensure that clean linen is used for each patient and that contaminated equipment is thoroughly cleaned. Routine cleaning schedules are also established to maintain hygiene standards (BMC Health Services Research, 2020).
5. **Needles and Syringes**: Policies dictate the proper disposal of used needles and syringes to prevent injuries and infections. These policies ensure that disposal containers are managed appropriately

and that cleaning staff handle the disposal process safely (Health Research Policy and Systems, 2014).

Healthcare policies are structured frameworks designed to address specific issues within the healthcare system. They include several critical *elements* that ensure the policy is comprehensive and effective.

Problem Statement

The problem statement clearly defines the issue or problem that the policy aims to address. This element is crucial as it frames the context and scope of the policy, ensuring that all stakeholders understand the specific challenge being tackled (Centers for Disease Control and Prevention [CDC], 2021).

Goals and Objectives

Goals and objectives outline the desired outcomes or targets that the policy seeks to achieve. These should be specific, measurable, achievable, relevant, and time-bound (SMART) to provide clear direction and benchmarks for success (CDC, 2021).

Target Population

Identifying the target population is essential for tailoring the policy interventions to the specific needs of the group affected. This ensures that the policy is relevant and effective in addressing the unique characteristics and requirements of the population (Unger, Morales, & De Paepe, 2020).

Policy Interventions

Policy interventions describe the specific actions or strategies that will be implemented to address the problem and achieve the goals. These interventions should be evidence-based and designed to produce measurable improvements in the identified problem area (de Leeuw, Clavier, & Breton, 2014).

Implementation Plan

The implementation plan details the steps involved in putting the policy into effect, including timelines, responsibilities, and resource allocation. This plan ensures that there is a clear roadmap for action and that all necessary resources are identified and allocated appropriately (BMC Health Services Research, 2020).

Evaluation Plan

An evaluation plan specifies the methods and criteria that will be used to assess the effectiveness of the policy in achieving its objectives. This includes both process and outcome evaluations to measure the implementation fidelity and the impact of the policy (CDC, 2021).

References and sources of the policy

References cite the sources of information used to develop and support the policy. This ensures that the policy is grounded in credible evidence and best practices, enhancing its legitimacy and effectiveness (de Leeuw, Clavier, & Breton, 2014).

Procedures

Procedures in healthcare are detailed, step-by-step instructions that guide healthcare professionals in performing specific tasks. These procedures are based on organizational policies and are essential for ensuring consistency, safety, and quality in patient care (Unger, Morales, & De Paepe, 2020).

Characteristics of Healthcare Procedures

Healthcare procedures serve as the "recipe" for how tasks are accomplished within a healthcare setting. They provide specific directions on what needs to be done, when it should be done, and who is responsible for doing it. This structured approach helps in standardizing care and minimizing errors (Centers for Disease Control and Prevention [CDC], 2021).

Examples of Healthcare Procedures

1. **Administering Blood**: This procedure involves several critical steps, including verifying patient identity, matching blood type, and monitoring for adverse reactions. Proper administration of blood is crucial to prevent complications such as transfusion reactions (BMC Health Services Research, 2020).

2. **Inserting Tubes**: Procedures for inserting nasogastric or urinary catheters include steps for ensuring sterility, proper placement, and patient comfort. These procedures are vital for preventing infections and ensuring the correct placement of the tubes (Unger, Morales, & De Paepe, 2020).

3. **Administering Medication**: This includes oral, rectal, and intravenous administration. Each method has specific steps to ensure the correct dosage, timing, and monitoring for side effects. Accurate medication administration is essential for effective treatment and patient safety (de Leeuw, Clavier, & Breton, 2014).

4. **Administering Tube Feedings**: This procedure involves preparing the feeding solution, ensuring the correct placement of the feeding tube, and monitoring the patient for tolerance and complications. Proper tube feeding is critical for patients who cannot eat by mouth (CDC, 2021).

5. **Performing Suctioning**: Suctioning procedures are used to clear the airway of secretions. This involves using sterile techniques to prevent infections and ensuring that the suctioning is effective without causing trauma to the patient (BMC Health Services Research, 2020).

6. **Wound Care**: This includes cleaning, dressing, and monitoring wounds. Proper wound care procedures are essential for promoting healing and preventing infections. Steps include using sterile materials, applying appropriate dressings, and monitoring for signs of infection (Unger, Morales, & De Paepe, 2020).

Guidelines

Clinical guidelines are systematically developed statements that assist healthcare practitioners in making decisions about appropriate care for specific clinical circumstances. They are typically based on a synthesis of current evidence and are meant to guide clinical practice while allowing flexibility for individualized patient care. The development of these guidelines involves evaluating and integrating scientific research, clinical expertise, and patient values. According to Field and Lohr (1990), clinical guidelines can improve the quality of care, reduce variations in practice, and optimize the use of healthcare resources.

Characteristics and Purpose of Clinical Guidelines

Clinical guidelines are evidence-based and aim to outline the most effective interventions for particular conditions. Unlike clinical pathways, which may provide a step-by-step approach, guidelines offer recommendations that can be adapted based on the clinician's judgment and the patient's unique circumstances. The flexibility of guidelines allows for adjustments when standard treatments may not be suitable due to factors such as patient comorbidities, preferences, or access to resources.

Implementation in Different Disciplines

1. Cardiology

In cardiology, clinical guidelines are widely used to manage conditions such as hypertension, heart failure, and coronary artery disease. The American College of Cardiology (ACC) and the American Heart Association (AHA) provide joint guidelines for the management of hypertension, recommending lifestyle changes, pharmacotherapy, and regular monitoring (Whelton et al., 2018). For example, the guidelines suggest using angiotensin-converting enzyme inhibitors or beta-blockers as first-line treatments for patients with hypertension who have had a previous myocardial infarction. Additionally, the guidelines for the management of heart failure include recommendations for the use of diuretics, angiotensin receptor-neprilysin inhibitors (ARNIs), and lifestyle modifications, which are based on clinical trials demonstrating their efficacy in reducing morbidity and mortality (Yancy et al., 2017).

The American College of Cardiology (ACC) and the American Heart Association (AHA) provide guidelines for the management of conditions such as atrial fibrillation, heart failure, and hypertension. These guidelines are based on extensive research and clinical trials, offering recommendations on diagnosis, treatment, and management strategies (American College of Cardiology, 2023). For instance, the guidelines for managing atrial fibrillation include recommendations on the use of anticoagulants, rate control, and rhythm control strategies (January et al., 2019).

2. Dental Care

In dentistry, clinical guidelines help inform the management of oral health conditions and procedures. The American Dental Association (ADA) provides guidelines for the prevention of dental caries, emphasizing the use of fluoride treatments, dental sealants, and patient education on oral hygiene (Wright et al., 2014). Furthermore, guidelines for the management of dental patients who are on anticoagulant therapy recommend evaluating the risk of bleeding against the risk of thrombosis when considering dental procedures, and adjusting anticoagulant doses accordingly (Little et al., 2012). These guidelines guide dentists on when it may be necessary to alter medication regimens before surgical procedures to prevent excessive bleeding. The American Dental Association (ADA) provides guidelines on various aspects of dental care, including pain management, caries treatment, and antibiotic use. For example, the ADA's guidelines on managing acute dental pain recommend specific analgesics and dosages for different age groups and conditions (American Dental Association, 2021). Additionally, guidelines for the use of silver diamine fluoride in caries management provide evidence-based recommendations for its application and effectiveness (Horst et al., 2016).

3. Anesthesia

Clinical guidelines in anesthesiology focus on patient safety and the effective management of anesthesia-related risks. For instance, the American Society of Anesthesiologists (ASA) has developed guidelines for the management of the difficult airway, which provide an algorithmic approach to ensure patient safety during intubation and airway management (Apfelbaum et al., 2013). These guidelines recommend specific techniques such as awake intubation or the use of fiberoptic intubation devices in cases where a difficult airway is anticipated. In addition, preoperative fasting guidelines suggest fasting times for solids and liquids to minimize the risk of aspiration during anesthesia, which is evidence-based and has been shown to improve patient safety (Practice Guidelines for Preoperative Fasting, 2017).

4. Laboratory Medicine

Clinical guidelines in laboratory medicine are important for ensuring the appropriate use of diagnostic tests and the interpretation of results. The Clinical and Laboratory Standards Institute (CLSI) provides guidelines for the accuracy and precision of laboratory testing procedures, such as blood glucose monitoring and coagulation tests. For instance, guidelines for hemoglobin A1c testing in diabetic patients recommend specific laboratory methods and quality control measures to ensure reliable results that can be used to monitor long-term glycemic control (American Diabetes Association, 2018). Following these guidelines helps standardize laboratory practices and ensures that test results are reliable and actionable for patient care.

5. Surgery

In the surgical field, clinical guidelines are used to enhance patient outcomes and minimize the risk of complications. For example, the World Health Organization's (WHO) guidelines for surgical safety advocate the use of a surgical safety checklist, which includes preoperative, intraoperative, and postoperative steps to reduce surgical site infections, bleeding, and other complications (Haynes et al., 2009). Additionally, guidelines for antibiotic prophylaxis in surgery recommend the administration of antibiotics within a specific timeframe before incision to prevent postoperative infections, with recommendations tailored to different types of surgeries (Bratzler et al., 2013).

6. Public Health

Public health guidelines are developed to address population health issues and provide recommendations for disease prevention and health promotion. The World Health Organization (WHO) develops guidelines on various public health topics, such as immunization schedules and breastfeeding practices. These guidelines are based on systematic reviews of evidence and aim to improve health outcomes on a global scale (World Health Organization, 2020).

7. Primary Healthcare

In primary healthcare, clinical guidelines assist in managing common conditions and promoting preventive care. The American Academy of Family Physicians (AAFP) provides guidelines on a wide range of topics, including chronic disease management, preventive screenings, and immunizations. These guidelines help primary care providers deliver evidence-based care and improve patient outcomes (American Academy of Family Physicians, 2023).

8. Nursing

Nursing guidelines are designed to support nurses in delivering high-quality, evidence-based care. The American Nurses Association (ANA) and other organizations provide guidelines on various aspects of nursing practice, including patient safety, infection control, and chronic disease management. These guidelines help standardize nursing care and ensure that patients receive consistent and effective treatment (Evidence-Based Nursing, 2023).

9. Surgery

Surgical guidelines are essential for standardizing procedures and improving patient outcomes. The American College of Surgeons (ACS) and other organizations provide guidelines on various surgical practices. For example, guidelines for antimicrobial prophylaxis in surgery recommend specific antibiotics and dosages to prevent surgical site infections (Bratzler et al., 2013). These guidelines are based on evidence from clinical trials and expert consensus, ensuring that patients receive the best possible care.

10. Healthcare Administration

In healthcare administration, guidelines help manage the organization and delivery of healthcare services. These guidelines cover areas such as quality improvement, patient safety, and healthcare policy. For example, the National Center for Complementary and Integrative Health (NCCIH) provides guidelines on the integration of complementary therapies into conventional healthcare practices (National Center for Complementary and Integrative Health, 2023).

Evidence Supporting Clinical Guidelines

The adoption of clinical guidelines has been shown to improve patient outcomes across various medical disciplines. For instance, a systematic review by Grimshaw et al. (2004) concluded that the use of clinical guidelines significantly enhances clinical practice by reducing variations in care and improving adherence to evidence-based practices. Another study by Cabana et al. (1999) highlighted that clinical guidelines improve healthcare outcomes when they are properly implemented and supported by educational interventions and organizational changes.

Guidelines are often updated based on new research findings, ensuring that healthcare providers have access to the latest evidence-based recommendations. This process involves a thorough review of new data, expert consensus, and patient preferences, making guidelines dynamic and adaptable to advancements in medical knowledge.

Clinical pathways

Clinical pathways, also known as critical pathways or care pathways, represent a structured approach to the delivery of healthcare for specific clinical diagnoses. They provide a detailed, day-by-day guide to standardized care, outlining the key interventions, anticipated timelines, and expected outcomes throughout a patient's course of treatment. The development and utilization of clinical pathways aim to enhance the quality of patient care, improve outcomes, and promote efficient use of healthcare resources by reducing variations in treatment and ensuring consistency in the management of similar patient groups.

Characteristics and Purpose of Clinical Pathways

Clinical pathways are multidisciplinary tools, involving the coordinated efforts of various healthcare professionals such as physicians, nurses, therapists, and other allied health staff. Their collaborative approach ensures that all care providers follow a unified plan, which integrates routine interventions and standard practices. Pathways are often created based on best practice guidelines and evidence from clinical studies, and they serve as a framework for decision-making across different phases of patient care. According to Vanhaecht et al. (2010), the main goal of clinical pathways is to improve the continuity and coordination of care for patients with specific diagnoses, ensuring that treatments are administered in a timely and appropriate manner. This standardized approach is beneficial in enhancing patient outcomes while optimizing the use of healthcare resources.

Implementation in Different healthcare specialties

1. Orthopedics

In orthopedic surgery, clinical pathways are frequently used to manage postoperative care for joint replacement surgeries such as total hip or knee arthroplasty. A study by Bozic et al. (2012) illustrated that the implementation of clinical pathways for hip replacement patients significantly reduced the length of hospital stays and improved pain management, while maintaining low complication rates. The pathway typically includes preoperative patient education, pain control protocols, early mobilization strategies, and scheduled physiotherapy sessions. The clinical pathway is designed to standardize postoperative care, reduce complications such as deep vein thrombosis, and facilitate quicker patient recovery (Bozic et al., 2012).

2. Oncology

Clinical pathways in oncology help manage chemotherapy regimens and monitor cancer treatment progress. According to Neuss et al. (2016), the use of standardized oncology clinical pathways has demonstrated an improvement in the consistency of care and a reduction in treatment-related costs. For example, patients with non-small cell lung cancer may follow a pathway that specifies diagnostic imaging, chemotherapy cycles, supportive care interventions such as anti-nausea medications, and periodic reassessment of tumor response. Clinical pathways provide a structured approach to cancer treatment, ensuring that care aligns with the latest clinical guidelines and evidence-based practices, which helps to enhance survival rates and quality of life for patients (Neuss et al., 2016).

3. Cardiology

In the management of acute myocardial infarction (AMI), clinical pathways are used to standardize the approach to interventions such as thrombolytic therapy, percutaneous coronary intervention (PCI), and post-acute care rehabilitation. A study by Cannon et al. (2002) indicated that using a clinical pathway for AMI management resulted in quicker administration of thrombolytics and a shorter time to cardiac catheterization, leading to improved patient outcomes. The pathway may involve steps such as immediate administration of aspirin, anticoagulants, and beta-blockers, followed by invasive procedures based on the patient's condition, thus streamlining the treatment process and improving survival rates (Cannon et al., 2002).

Integration of Clinical Standards and Performance Criteria

Clinical pathways are designed to incorporate clinical standards and performance benchmarks, which are measurable outcomes or quality indicators used to assess the efficacy of the care provided. They often include key performance indicators (KPIs) such as the time to initiate treatment, length of stay, readmission rates, and complication rates. These criteria help to evaluate whether the planned interventions are achieving the desired clinical outcomes within the specified time frames.

According to Rotter et al. (2010), clinical pathways effectively reduce variability in care processes and enhance patient outcomes when they are implemented alongside performance criteria. For instance, in the case of stroke rehabilitation, pathways may include performance criteria related to mobility milestones, cognitive function, and daily living activities. This integration ensures that clinical care adheres to established standards while allowing for ongoing monitoring and adjustment of interventions as needed.

Evidence Supporting the Use of Clinical Pathways

Several systematic reviews and meta-analyses have supported the efficacy of clinical pathways in improving patient outcomes. A meta-analysis by Allen et al. (2009) found that the implementation of clinical pathways significantly reduced hospital costs, shortened the length of stay, and improved clinical outcomes in patients undergoing various surgical procedures. Similarly, a systematic review by Rotter et al. (2010) demonstrated that clinical pathways were associated with a reduction in in-hospital complications and mortality rates in multiple disciplines, including orthopedics, cardiology, and general surgery.

The pathways are particularly beneficial in settings where care delivery involves complex processes requiring the coordination of multiple healthcare providers. By establishing a standardized approach to care, clinical pathways help to streamline workflow, reduce the likelihood of errors, and ensure that patients receive timely and appropriate interventions.

Protocols

Protocol: A protocol is a stringent, detailed, and planned process for managing a clinical condition. For example, the World Health Organization (WHO) has established protocols for the management of diarrhea cases. These protocols include the use of Oral Rehydration Salts (ORS) and zinc supplements to reduce the duration and severity of diarrheal episodes (World Health Organization, 2005).

Post-Operative Care Protocol (First 24 Hours)

Expected Outcome: The patient will recover from the surgical procedure without experiencing complications (American Society of Anesthesiologists, 2013).

Interventions

1. **Bed Rest**: The patient should remain in bed and be turned every two hours to prevent pressure sores and improve circulation (Pearsall et al., 2017).
2. **Ice Chips Only**: Provide ice chips to the patient and assess for nausea and vomiting (Pearsall et al., 2017).
3. **Urine Output**: Check urine output every hour for the first 12 hours. It should be 30cc/hour or greater (Pearsall et al., 2017).
4. **IV Fluids**: Monitor intravenous fluids and assess the IV site every 12 hours (Pearsall et al., 2017).
5. **Bowel Sounds**: Assess for bowel sounds every 8 hours to ensure normal gastrointestinal function (Pearsall et al., 2017).
6. **Deep Breathing**: Encourage the patient to take deep breaths every two hours to prevent atelectasis (Pearsall et al., 2017).
7. **Lung Assessment**: Assess the patient's lungs every 12 hours to monitor for respiratory complications (Pearsall et al., 2017).
8. **Skin Assessment**: Check the color and warmth of the patient's skin every 8 hours to detect any circulatory issues (Pearsall et al., 2017).

9. **Surgical Dressing**: Assess the surgical dressing upon admission to the ward and then every 4 hours to monitor for signs of infection or excessive bleeding (Pearsall et al., 2017).
10. **Pain Relief**: Assess the patient's need for pain relief and medicate as indicated (Pearsall et al., 2017).
11. **Patient and Family Education**: Explain to the patient and their family what they can expect regarding care and treatment during the recovery period (Pearsall et al., 2017).

Standard Operating Procedures (SOPs)

SOP: A Standard Operating Procedure (SOP) is a statement of the expected way in which an organization's staff carries out certain activities. SOPs provide detailed, written instructions to achieve uniformity in the performance of specific functions. For example, an SOP for billing patients would outline the steps to be followed to ensure accurate and consistent billing practices (American Society for Quality, 2020).

SOPs in Healthcare

Definition and Purpose: SOPs provide instructions on how to proceed under specific circumstances. They are administrative actions rather than technical actions. For instance, if a medication error has been made, an SOP would describe what to report, to whom, and the steps to follow to address the error (Joint Commission, 2019).

Example SOP: Medication Error

When a medication error occurs, the person discovering the error will:

1. **Notify the Prescribing Physician**: Immediately inform the prescribing physician about the error.
2. **Complete a Medication Occurrence Report**: Document the error in a medication occurrence report.
3. **Signatures**: Have the unit manager and director sign the report.
4. **Documentation in Patient's Chart**: Record all medications given to the patient in their chart. If an explanation for an omission is apparent

(e.g., the patient was away from the nursing unit for tests), document that reason in the record.

5. **Notify the Pharmacist**: Inform the pharmacist if the error involves the pharmacy (Institute for Safe Medication Practices, 2021).

Follow-Up Actions

- **Trending and Reporting**: All medication errors and potential errors are trended and reported to the pharmacy committee quarterly. Serious medication errors are summarized and reviewed by the pharmacy committee, including severity level/outcome classifications.

- **Manager's Role**: The manager of the area where the medication error occurred will determine the appropriate follow-up actions based on the seriousness of the errors and document the action plan. The intent of the action plan is for education rather than punishment.

- **Consultation for Serious Errors**: In case of a serious prescribing error, the chairman of the pharmacy committee will consult with the chairman of the medical department of the physician involved (Joint Commission, 2019).

Healthcare Standards

Standards Defined: Standards (criteria) are statements of expectations for the structure, processes, and outcomes of the healthcare system that are necessary to ensure the delivery of quality patient care (Joint Commission, 2019).

Characteristics of Standards

1. **Valid**: Standards must be based on sound evidence and best practices.
2. **Reliable**: They should produce consistent results when applied in similar contexts.
3. **Clear**: Standards need to be easily understood and unambiguous.
4. **Applicable**: They must be relevant and practical for the intended setting (World Health Organization, 2018).

Functions of Standards

- **Operational Translation**: Standards translate quality into operational terms and hold everyone in the system accountable.
- **Measurement**: They allow organizations to measure quality levels.
- **Consistency**: Standards encourage consistency and uniformity in healthcare delivery (Institute of Medicine, 2001).

Why Standards?

- **Variation**: To reduce variability in healthcare practices.
- **Payment Reimbursement and Litigation Requirements**: Standards help meet the requirements for reimbursement and protect against litigation.
- **Licensing**: They are often required for licensing and accreditation purposes (National Institute for Health and Care Excellence, 2019).

Healthcare Algorithms

Healthcare algorithms are systematic, step-by-step procedures or formulas used to make clinical decisions and solve medical problems. These algorithms are designed to improve the accuracy and efficiency of healthcare delivery by providing clear guidelines for diagnosis, treatment, and management of various health conditions.

Definition and Purpose

Healthcare algorithms are essential tools in clinical practice. They help standardize care, reduce variability, and ensure that patients receive evidence-based treatments. Algorithms can range from simple decision trees to complex computational models that integrate multiple data sources (Topol, 2019).

Types of Healthcare Algorithms

1. **Diagnostic Algorithms**: These algorithms assist healthcare providers in diagnosing diseases based on patient symptoms, medical history, and test results. For example, the algorithm for diagnosing diabetes includes

steps such as measuring fasting blood glucose levels and conducting an oral glucose tolerance test (American Diabetes Association, 2020).

2. **Treatment Algorithms**: These provide step-by-step instructions for treating specific conditions. For instance, the American Heart Association's algorithm for managing acute coronary syndrome outlines the use of medications, lifestyle changes, and surgical interventions (American Heart Association, 2019).

3. **Prognostic Algorithms**: These predict the likely outcomes of diseases and help in planning patient care. An example is the use of the APACHE II score to predict mortality in critically ill patients (Knaus et al., 1985).

4. **Management Algorithms**: These guide the overall management of chronic diseases, including monitoring and follow-up care. The algorithm for managing hypertension includes regular blood pressure monitoring, lifestyle modifications, and medication adjustments (National Institute for Health and Care Excellence, 2019).

Benefits of Healthcare Algorithms

Healthcare algorithms offer several benefits, including:

- **Improved Decision-Making**: By providing evidence-based guidelines, algorithms help clinicians make more accurate and consistent decisions (Topol, 2019).
- **Efficiency**: Algorithms streamline the diagnostic and treatment processes, reducing the time and resources needed for patient care (American Diabetes Association, 2020).
- **Patient Outcomes**: The use of algorithms has been shown to improve patient outcomes by ensuring timely and appropriate interventions (American Heart Association, 2019).

Challenges and Limitations

Despite their benefits, healthcare algorithms also face challenges:

- **Complexity**: Some algorithms are complex and require significant training to use effectively (Topol, 2019).

- **Data Quality**: The accuracy of algorithms depends on the quality of the data used to develop them. Poor data quality can lead to incorrect recommendations (Knaus et al., 1985).
- **Ethical Concerns**: The use of algorithms raises ethical issues, such as patient privacy and the potential for bias in algorithmic decision-making (National Institute for Health and Care Excellence, 2019).

Table 5.1: Summary of health directives

Term	Definition	Purpose	Example
Policies	Broad statements that outline an organization's intentions and direction.	Provide a framework for decision-making and ensure consistency.	Hospital policy on patient confidentiality.
Procedures	Detailed, step-by-step instructions on how to perform specific tasks.	Ensure tasks are performed correctly and consistently.	Procedure for administering medication.
Pathways	Structured multidisciplinary care plans detailing essential steps in patient care.	Optimize patient outcomes and streamline care processes.	Clinical pathway for managing stroke patients.
Guidelines	Systematically developed statements to assist practitioner and patient decisions.	Provide evidence-based recommendations for clinical practice.	WHO guidelines for the treatment of tuberculosis.
Protocols	Stringent, detailed, and planned processes for managing specific clinical conditions.	Ensure specific clinical conditions are managed effectively and consistently.	WHO protocols for diarrhea case management.
Algorithms	Step-by-step problem-solving processes or rules to be followed in calculations or other	Provide a clear method for solving problems or performing tasks.	Algorithm for diagnosing diabetes.

Term	Definition	Purpose	Example
	problem-solving operations.		
SOPs	Standard Operating Procedures; detailed written instructions to achieve uniformity.	Ensure consistency and quality in performing specific functions.	SOP for sterilizing surgical instruments.
Standards	Established norms or requirements about technical systems and practices.	Ensure safety, quality, and efficiency in healthcare services.	ISO standards for healthcare quality management systems.

To simplify these terms, an example of dental abscess to illustrate each term discussed in this chapter:

- **Policies**: These are like the rules of the dental clinic. For example, the clinic policy might state that all patients with signs of a dental abscess must be evaluated immediately to ensure timely treatment.
- **Procedures**: These are the step-by-step instructions for specific tasks. For instance, the procedure for draining a dental abscess includes steps like sterilizing the area, making an incision, and draining the pus.
- **Pathways**: These are detailed plans for specific patient care situations. For example, the clinical pathway for a dental abscess would outline all the steps from the initial assessment, through treatment, to follow-up care, including pain management and antibiotics.
- **Guidelines**: These are tips and advice on the best ways to provide care. For example, guidelines for managing a dental abscess might recommend the use of specific antibiotics and pain relief methods, as well as advice on oral hygiene to prevent future abscesses.
- **Protocols**: These are strict rules for specific medical scenarios. For instance, the protocol for handling a severe dental abscess might include immediate incision and drainage, administration of intravenous antibiotics, and close monitoring of the patient's vital signs.
- **Algorithms**: These are like flowcharts that help healthcare providers decide what to do next. For example, an algorithm for diagnosing a

dental abscess might include steps like checking for symptoms (e.g., swelling, pain), performing a physical examination, and ordering imaging tests if necessary.

- **SOPs (Standard Operating Procedures)**: These are detailed instructions to ensure everyone performs tasks the same way. For example, an SOP for sterilizing dental instruments would include specific steps to clean, disinfect, and store the instruments properly.
- **Standards**: These are the criteria that define what makes good dental care. For example, standards for treating dental abscesses ensure that all patients receive timely and effective care to prevent complications and promote healing.

Another example to explain these terms the COVID 19 pandemic to illustrate each term:

- **Policies**: These are like the rules of the public health department. For example, a policy might state that all confirmed COVID-19 cases must be reported to the health department within 24 hours to ensure timely response and containment.
- **Procedures**: These are the step-by-step instructions for specific tasks. For instance, the procedure for testing a patient for COVID-19 includes steps like collecting a nasal swab sample, processing the sample in a lab, and reporting the results.
- **Pathways**: These are detailed plans for specific public health situations. For example, the pathway for managing a COVID-19 patient would outline all the steps from initial testing, through treatment and isolation, to follow-up care and contact tracing.
- **Guidelines**: These are tips and advice on the best ways to manage public health issues. For example, guidelines for managing COVID-19 might recommend social distancing, mask-wearing, and vaccination to reduce transmission.
- **Protocols**: These are strict rules for specific public health scenarios. For instance, the protocol for handling a severe COVID-19 outbreak might include immediate lockdown measures, administration of antiviral medications, and activation of emergency response teams.

- **Algorithms**: These are like flowcharts that help public health professionals decide what to do next. For example, an algorithm for diagnosing COVID-19 might include steps like checking for symptoms (e.g., fever, cough), performing a PCR test, and confirming the diagnosis with additional tests if necessary.
- **SOPs (Standard Operating Procedures)**: These are detailed instructions to ensure everyone performs tasks the same way. For example, an SOP for administering COVID-19 vaccines would include specific steps to prepare the vaccine, administer it safely, and monitor for adverse reactions.
- **Standards**: These are the criteria that define what makes good public health practice. For example, standards for managing COVID-19 ensure that all public health actions are timely, effective, and based on the best available evidence to protect the population.

References

1. Allen, D., Gillen, E., & Rixson, L. (2009). Systematic review of the effectiveness of integrated care pathways: What works, for whom, in which circumstances? International Journal of Evidence-Based Healthcare, 7(2), 61-74. https://doi.org/10.1111/j.1744-1609.2009.00127.x

2. American College of Cardiology. (2023). Guidelines & Clinical Documents. https://www.acc.org/guidelines

3. American Dental Association. (2021). Clinical Practice Guidelines and Dental Evidence. https://www.ada.org/resources/research/science-and-research-institute/evidence-based-dental-research

4. American Diabetes Association. (2020). Standards of medical care in diabetes---2020 abridged for primary care providers. Clinical Diabetes, 38(1), 10-38. https://doi.org/10.2337/cd20-as01

5. American Heart Association. (2019). 2019 AHA/ACC guideline on the primary prevention of cardiovascular disease: A report of the American College of Cardiology/American Heart Association Task Force on Clinical Practice Guidelines. Circulation, 140(11), e596-e646. https://doi.org/10.1161/CIR.0000000000000678

6. American Society of Anesthesiologists. (2017). Practice Guidelines for Preoperative Fasting and the Use of Pharmacologic Agents to Reduce the Risk of Pulmonary Aspiration. Anesthesiology, 126(3), 376-393. https://pubs.asahq.org/anesthesiology/article/126/3/376/19732/Practice-Guidelines-for-Preoperative-Fasting-and

7. Apfelbaum, J. L., Hagberg, C. A., Caplan, R. A., Blitt, C. D., Connis, R. T., Nickinovich, D. G., & Benumof, J. L. (2013). Practice guidelines for management of the difficult airway: An updated report by the American Society of Anesthesiologists Task Force on Management of the Difficult Airway. Anesthesiology, 118(2), 251-270. https://doi.org/10.1097/ALN.0b013e31827773b2

8. Bozic, K. J., Wagie, A., & Naessens, J. M. (2012). The impact of clinical pathway implementation on the quality of life in patients undergoing total hip arthroplasty. Journal of Bone and Joint Surgery, 94(22), 2041-2047. https://doi.org/10.2106/JBJS.K.01239

9. Bratzler, D. W., Dellinger, E. P., Olsen, K. M., Perl, T. M., Auwaerter, P. G., Bolon, M. K., ... & Fish, D. N. (2013). Clinical practice guidelines for antimicrobial prophylaxis in surgery. American Journal of Health-System Pharmacy, 70(3), 195-283. https://academic.oup.com/ajhp/article/70/3/195/5113379

10. Cabana, M. D., Rand, C. S., Powe, N. R., Wu, A. W., Wilson, M. H., Abboud, P. A., & Rubin, H. R. (1999). Why don't physicians follow clinical practice guidelines? A framework for improvement. JAMA, 282(15), 1458-1465. https://doi.org/10.1001/jama.282.15.1458

11. Cannon, C. P., Gibson, C. M., Lambrew, C. T., & French, W. J. (2002). Relationship of symptom-onset-to-balloon time and door-to-balloon time with mortality in patients undergoing angioplasty for acute myocardial infarction. Journal of the American College of Cardiology, 40(9), 1579-1585. https://doi.org/10.1016/S0735-1097(02)02272-5

12. Centers for Disease Control and Prevention. (2021). Roles in the CDC policy process. https://www.cdc.gov/polaris/php/policy-resources-trainings/roles-in-the-cdc-policy-process.html

13. .Clinical and Laboratory Standards Institute. (2020). Performance Standards for Antimicrobial Susceptibility Testing. https://clsi.org/standards/products/microbiology/documents/m100/

14. De Leeuw, E., Clavier, C., & Breton, E. (2014). Health policy -- why research it and how: health political science. Health Research Policy and Systems, 12, Article 55. https://health-policy-systems.biomedcentral.com/articles/10.1186/1478-4505-12-55

15. Evidence-Based Nursing. (2023). Clinical practice guidelines. https://ebn.bmj.com/content/2/2/38

16. Field, M. J., & Lohr, K. N. (Eds.). (1990). Clinical practice guidelines: Directions for a new program. National Academies Press.

17. Grimshaw, J. M., Thomas, R. E., MacLennan, G., Fraser, C., Ramsay, C. R., Vale, L., & Donaldson, C. (2004). Effectiveness and efficiency of guideline dissemination and implementation strategies. Health Technology Assessment, 8(6), 1-72. https://doi.org/10.3310/hta8060

18. Haynes, A. B., Weiser, T. G., Berry, W. R., Lipsitz, S. R., Breizat, A. H. S., Dellinger, E. P., & Gawande, A. A. (2009). A surgical safety checklist to reduce morbidity and mortality in a global population. New England Journal of Medicine, 360(5), 491-499. https://doi.org/10.1056/NEJMsa0810119

19. Horst, J. A., Ellenikiotis, H., & Milgrom, P. L. (2016). UCSF Protocol for Caries Arrest Using Silver Diamine Fluoride: Rationale, Indications, and Consent. Journal of the California Dental Association, 44(1), 16-28. https://pubmed. ncbi.nlm.nih.gov/26897901/

20. Institute of Medicine. (2001). Crossing the quality chasm: A new health system for the 21st century. National Academies Press. https://doi.org/10.17226/10027

21. January, C. T., Wann, L. S., Calkins, H., Chen, L. Y., Cigarroa, J. E., Cleveland, J. C., ... & Yancy, C. W. (2019). 2019 AHA/ACC/HRS focused update of the 2014 AHA/ACC/HRS guideline for the management of patients with atrial fibrillation. Journal of the American College of Cardiology, 74(1), 104-132. https://www.jacc.org/doi/10.1016/j.jacc.2019.01.011

22. Joint Commission. (2019). Comprehensive Accreditation Manual for Hospitals (CAMH). Joint Commission Resources. https://www.jointcommission.org/standards_information/standards.aspx

23. Knaus, W. A., Draper, E. A., Wagner, D. P., & Zimmerman, J. E. (1985). APACHE II: A severity of disease classification system. Critical Care Medicine, 13(10), 818-829. https://doi.org/10.1097/00003246-198510000-00009

24. Little, J. W., Miller, C. S., & Rhodus, N. L. (2012). Dental management of the medically compromised patient. Elsevier Health Sciences.

25. National Center for Complementary and Integrative Health. (2023). Clinical Practice Guidelines. https://www.nccih.nih.gov/health/providers/clinicalpractice

26. National Institute for Health and Care Excellence. (2019). Hypertension in adults: Diagnosis and management (NICE Guideline NG136). https://www.nice.org.uk/guidance/ng136

27. Neuss, M. N., Polovich, M., McNiff, K., Esper, P., Gilmore, T. R., LeFebvre, K. B., & Jacobson, J. O. (2016). Updated American Society of Clinical Oncology/Oncology Nursing Society chemotherapy administration safety standards, including standards for pediatric oncology. Journal of Oncology Practice, 12(12), 1262-1271. https://doi.org/10.1200/JOP.2016.017905

28. Pearsall, E., McCluskey, S., Aarts, M. A., & McLeod, R. (2017). Enhanced Recovery after Surgery: ERAS for All. Best Practice in Surgery, University of Toronto. http://bestpracticeinsurgery.ca/wp-content/uploads/2017/11/ERAS_BPS_FINAL_Nov2017.pdf

29. Rotter, T., Kinsman, L., James, E., Machotta, A., Willis, J., Snow, P., & Kugler, J. (2010). Clinical pathways: Effects on professional practice, patient outcomes, length of stay and hospital costs. Cochrane Database of Systematic Reviews, 3(3), CD006632. https://doi.org/10.1002/14651858.CD006632.pub2

30. Topol, E. (2019). Deep medicine: How artificial intelligence can make healthcare human again. Basic Books.

31. Unger, J. P., Morales, I., & De Paepe, P. (2020). Objectives, methods, and results in critical health systems and policy research: evaluating the healthcare market. BMC Health Services Research, 20, Article 1072. https://bmchealthservres.biomedcentral.com/articles/10.1186/s12913-020-05889-w

32. Vanhaecht, K., Panella, M., van Zelm, R., & Sermeus, W. (2010). An overview on the history and concept of care pathways as complex interventions. International Journal of Care Pathways, 14(3), 117-123. https://doi.org/10.1258/jicp.2010.010019

33. Whelton, P. K., Carey, R. M., Aronow, W. S., Casey, D. E., Collins, K. J., Himmelfarb, C. D., & Wright, J. T. (2018). 2017 ACC/AHA/AAPA/ABC/ACPM/AGS/APhA/ASH/ASPC/NMA/PCNA guideline for the prevention, detection, evaluation, and management of high blood pressure in adults. Journal of the American College of Cardiology, 71(19), e127-e248. https://doi.org/10.1016/j.jacc.2017.11.006

34. World Health Organization. (2018). Standards for improving quality of maternal and newborn care in health facilities. https://www.who.int/maternal_child_adolescent/documents/improving-maternal-newborn-care-quality/en/

35. Wright, J. T., Crall, J. J., Fontana, M., Gillette, E. J., Nový, B. B., Dhar, V., & Berg, J. H. (2014). Evidence-based clinical practice guideline for the use of pit-and-fissure sealants: A report of the American Dental Association and the American Academy of Pediatric Dentistry. Journal of the American Dental Association, 145(8), 835-849. https://doi.org/10.142

Chapter 6

Quality Performance Measures

Healthcare quality performance measures are essential tools used to evaluate the effectiveness, efficiency, and equity of healthcare services. These measures are critical for ensuring that healthcare systems deliver high-quality care that meets the needs of patients and improves overall health outcomes. According to Donabedian (1988), healthcare quality can be assessed through three primary dimensions: structure, process, and outcome. Each of these dimensions provides a unique perspective on the quality of care and helps identify areas for improvement.

Purpose of Performance Measures

Performance measures are vital tools in healthcare that help evaluate the quality of care provided by healthcare organizations. These measures are essential for several reasons:

1. **Improving Patient Outcomes**: By systematically measuring performance, healthcare providers can identify areas where patient care can be improved. This leads to better health outcomes, such as reduced mortality rates, fewer complications, and enhanced patient satisfaction (Donabedian, 1988; IBM, 2023).
2. **Ensuring Accountability**: Performance measures hold healthcare providers accountable for the quality of care they deliver. This accountability is crucial for maintaining trust between patients and

healthcare providers, as well as between healthcare organizations and regulatory bodies (Donabedian, 1988; Joint Commission, 2023).

3. **Facilitating Continuous Improvement**: Regular measurement and analysis of performance data enable healthcare organizations to implement continuous quality improvement initiatives. These initiatives can lead to more efficient processes, reduced errors, and better resource utilization (Donabedian, 1988; American Academy of Family Physicians, 2023).

4. **Supporting Evidence-Based Practice**: Performance measures help ensure that healthcare practices are based on the best available evidence. By adhering to established guidelines and protocols, healthcare providers can deliver care that is both effective and consistent (Donabedian, 1988; IBM, 2023).

5. **Enhancing Patient Safety**: Measuring performance helps identify potential safety issues before they result in harm. This proactive approach to patient safety can prevent adverse events and improve the overall safety of healthcare environments (Donabedian, 1988; Joint Commission, 2023).

6. **Informing Policy and Decision-Making**: Performance data provide valuable insights for policymakers and healthcare leaders. These insights can inform decisions about resource allocation, policy development, and strategic planning, ultimately leading to a more effective and efficient healthcare system (Donabedian, 1988; Continu, 2023).

Key Performance Indicators (KPIs) in Healthcare Quality

Definition and Purpose of KPIs

Key Performance Indicators (KPIs) are specific, quantifiable measures used to evaluate the performance of healthcare services. They provide a clear and objective way to assess various aspects of healthcare quality, including clinical outcomes, patient satisfaction, and operational efficiency (Databox, 2023; Insightsoftware, 2024).

Evolution of Performance Measures in Healthcare

Brief History and Development of Performance Measurement Practices

The concept of performance measurement in healthcare has evolved significantly over the past century. Early efforts can be traced back to the early 20th century when Dr. Ernest Codman introduced the "End Result Idea," advocating for tracking patient outcomes to improve care quality (Codman, 1914). This idea laid the groundwork for systematic performance measurement in healthcare.

In the mid-20th century, the principles of quality management from manufacturing, such as those developed by W. Edwards Deming, Joseph Juran, and Philip Crosby, began to influence healthcare. These principles emphasized continuous improvement, reducing variation, and focusing on customer satisfaction (Deming, 1986; Juran, 1988; Crosby, 1979).

The 1990s saw significant advancements with the establishment of organizations like the National Committee for Quality Assurance (NCQA) and the introduction of the Healthcare Effectiveness Data and Information Set (HEDIS), which provided standardized performance measures for health plans (NCQA, 1997). Around the same time, the Institute of Medicine (IOM) published influential reports such as "To Err is Human" (1999) and "Crossing the Quality Chasm" (2001), which highlighted the need for robust performance measurement to improve patient safety and healthcare quality (IOM, 1999; IOM, 2001).

Milestones in Quality and Performance Measurement in Healthcare

1. **1950s-1980s**: Adoption of quality management principles from manufacturing (Deming, 1986; Juran, 1988; Crosby, 1979).
2. **1990**: Establishment of the National Committee for Quality Assurance (NCQA).
3. **1997**: Introduction of the Healthcare Effectiveness Data and Information Set (HEDIS) by NCQA (NCQA, 1997).
4. **1999**: Publication of "To Err is Human" by the Institute of Medicine (IOM, 1999).

5. **2001**: Publication of "Crossing the Quality Chasm" by the Institute of Medicine (IOM, 2001).
6. **2005**: Introduction of Performance-Improvement Continuing Medical Education (PI-CME) by the American Medical Association (AMA, 2005).
7. **2010s**: Increased use of electronic health records (EHRs) and clinical registries to enhance performance measurement (Wiley, 2015).

Types of performance measures according to the Donabedian Model

Structure measures refer to the attributes of the settings in which care occurs. These include the physical and organizational infrastructure, such as facilities, equipment, and human resources (Donabedian, 1988). For example, the availability of advanced medical technology and the qualifications of healthcare professionals are key structural components that can influence the quality of care provided (Donabedian, 1988).

Process measures focus on the methods by which healthcare is delivered. These measures assess whether the care provided is consistent with current professional knowledge and guidelines (Donabedian, 1988). Examples of process measures include adherence to clinical protocols, timeliness of care, and the accuracy of diagnostic procedures. Process measures are crucial for ensuring that patients receive appropriate and effective treatments (Donabedian, 1988).

Outcome measures evaluate the results of healthcare services on the health status of patients. These measures include clinical outcomes, such as mortality and morbidity rates, as well as patient-reported outcomes, such as satisfaction and quality of life (Donabedian, 1988). Outcome measures are vital for assessing the ultimate impact of healthcare interventions on patient health and well-being (Donabedian, 1988).

Types of Healthcare KPIs

Clinical Quality KPIs

Clinical Quality KPIs are metrics that measure the effectiveness of clinical care. These include indicators such as mortality rates, infection rates, and readmission rates. Monitoring these KPIs helps healthcare providers identify areas where clinical practices can be improved to enhance patient outcomes (Databox, 2023; Insightsoftware, 2024).

Patient Safety KPIs

Patient Safety KPIs focus on the safety of patients within healthcare settings. These include incident reports, adverse events, and medication errors. Tracking these KPIs is crucial for identifying potential safety issues and implementing measures to prevent harm to patients (Databox, 2023; Insightsoftware, 2024).

Operational Efficiency KPIs

Operational Efficiency KPIs measure the efficiency of healthcare operations. Examples include wait times, length of stay, and occupancy rates. These KPIs help healthcare organizations optimize their processes to improve service delivery and reduce costs (Databox, 2023; Insightsoftware, 2024).

Patient Experience and Satisfaction KPIs

Patient Experience and Satisfaction KPIs assess the quality of the patient experience. These include HCAHPS scores and patient satisfaction surveys. High scores in these KPIs indicate that patients are satisfied with the care they receive, which is essential for patient retention and positive health outcomes (Databox, 2023; Insightsoftware, 2024).

Financial Performance KPIs

Financial Performance KPIs evaluate the financial health of healthcare organizations. These include cost per discharge, revenue growth, and billing accuracy. Monitoring these KPIs ensures that healthcare providers are financially sustainable while delivering high-quality care (Databox, 2023; Insightsoftware, 2024).

Workforce/Staff KPIs

Workforce/Staff KPIs measure aspects related to the healthcare workforce. These include staff turnover rate, training completion rates, and staff satisfaction. These KPIs are important for maintaining a skilled and motivated workforce, which is critical for delivering high-quality patient care (Databox, 2023; Insightsoftware, 2024).

Criteria for Selecting KPIs in Healthcare:

Selecting the right Key Performance Indicators (KPIs) in healthcare is crucial for ensuring that performance measurement aligns with organizational goals and improves healthcare quality. Here are the key criteria for selecting KPIs:

Relevance to Organizational Goals: KPIs should directly relate to the strategic objectives of the healthcare organization. This ensures that the performance measures are aligned with the overall mission and vision of the organization (Databox, 2023). For example, if a hospital aims to improve patient safety, relevant KPIs might include the rate of hospital-acquired infections or medication errors.

Stakeholder Input and Regulatory Requirements: Involving stakeholders, including healthcare providers, patients, and regulatory bodies, in the selection process ensures that the KPIs are comprehensive and address the needs and expectations of all parties involved (HIQA, 2013). Regulatory requirements often mandate specific KPIs to ensure compliance with national healthcare standards (Insightsoftware, 2024).

Alignment with Evidence-Based Standards and Benchmarks: KPIs should be based on evidence-based practices and aligned with national or international benchmarks. This helps in comparing performance against established standards and identifying areas for improvement (HIQA, 2013). For instance, using benchmarks from the National Committee for

Quality Assurance (NCQA) can provide a standard for evaluating clinical quality (NCQA, 1997).

KPI Development Process:

Developing effective KPIs involves several steps to ensure they are relevant, reliable, and actionable:

Identification: The first step is to identify potential KPIs that align with the organization's goals and objectives. This involves reviewing existing performance data, consulting with stakeholders, and considering regulatory requirements (Cascade Strategy, 2023).

Validation: Once potential KPIs are identified, they need to be validated to ensure they accurately measure what they are intended to. This may involve statistical analysis and pilot testing to confirm their reliability and validity (KPI.org, 2023).

Pilot Testing: Before full deployment, KPIs should be pilot tested in a controlled environment. This helps identify any issues with data collection, measurement, or interpretation and allows for adjustments to be made (Cascade Strategy, 2023).

Deployment: After successful pilot testing, KPIs can be fully deployed across the organization. This involves integrating them into the organization's performance management system and ensuring that all relevant staff are trained on how to collect and use the data (KPI.org, 2023).

Role of Data Sources, Technology, and Stakeholder Engagement: Effective KPI development relies on accurate and timely data from reliable sources. Technology, such as electronic health records (EHRs) and data analytics tools, plays a crucial role in collecting and analyzing KPI data (Insightsoftware, 2024). Engaging stakeholders throughout the process ensures that the KPIs are relevant and actionable, and that there is buy-in from all parties involved (HIQA, 2013).

Why measure performance?

Measuring performance is crucial for several reasons. **Firstly**, it provides facts by which to manage. According to Spitzer (2007), effective measurement directs behavior, increases visibility of performance, and focuses attention. This aligns with the idea that people pay more attention to facts, which helps in making informed decisions (Spitzer, 2007).

Secondly, measurement helps in making decisions based on facts. As noted by Rice (2024), setting clear, measurable goals and expectations for each role and team in alignment with organizational objectives is vital. This ensures that decisions are grounded in objective data rather than subjective judgment (Rice, 2024).

Thirdly, measurement creates opportunities for improvement. Performance metrics can highlight areas needing enhancement, thus fostering continuous improvement (Rice, 2024). Additionally, recognizing successes through measurement can boost morale and motivation among employees (Rice, 2024).

Lastly, measurement is essential for evaluating performance. It provides a structured, data-driven approach to assess how well employees meet the specific requirements of their roles (Rice, 2024). This evaluation is critical for both individual and organizational growth.

Elements of an indicator:

When developing indicators for healthcare quality and patient safety, it is essential to include several key components to ensure clarity and effectiveness. Each indicator should have the following elements:

Title: The title should clearly and concisely describe what the indicator measures. For example, "Hospital-Acquired Infection Rate" or "Patient Satisfaction Score" (Agency for Healthcare Research and Quality [AHRQ], 2022).

Goal: The goal defines the purpose of the indicator and what it aims to achieve. For instance, the goal of the "Hospital-Acquired Infection Rate" indicator might be to "Reduce the incidence of infections acquired during hospital stays to improve patient outcomes and safety" (AHRQ, 2022).

Definition: This section provides a detailed explanation of what the indicator measures. For example, "Hospital-Acquired Infection Rate" could be defined as "the number of infections acquired by patients during their hospital stay per 1,000 patient days" (AHRQ, 2022).

Definition of Important Terms: Clarify any terms that are critical to understanding the indicator. For example, "infection" might be defined as "an invasion and multiplication of microorganisms such as bacteria, viruses, and parasites that are not normally present within the body" (Centers for Disease Control and Prevention [CDC], 2023).

Common Data Sources: Identify where the data for the indicator will come from. Common sources might include medical records, patient surveys, and administrative databases (AHRQ, 2022).

Recommended Data Collection Methods: Suggest the best methods for collecting data. For example, data for the "Hospital-Acquired Infection Rate" might be collected through regular reviews of patient medical records and infection control logs (AHRQ, 2022).

Use: Explain how the indicator will be used to inform decisions or actions. For example, the "Hospital-Acquired Infection Rate" might be used to identify areas needing improvement in infection control practices and to track the effectiveness of interventions implemented (AHRQ, 2022).

Recommended Format of Presentation: Describe how the data should be presented to stakeholders. This could include charts, graphs, or dashboards that make the information easy to understand and act upon (AHRQ, 2022).

Calculation methods of a KPI

Rate-based indicators:

Are essential tools in healthcare for monitoring various events or processes over time. These indicators are particularly useful for tracking occurrences such as Caesarian sections (C-sections), vaginal births after C-section (VBACs), unexpected deaths, and clean wound infections. One common example of a rate-based indicator is the readmission rate, which measures the frequency of patients being readmitted to a hospital within a specific period after discharge (Mainz, 2003).

Rate-based indicators measure the proportion of occurrences or events in relation to the population at risk. To determine the rate, the number of occurrences (numerator) is divided by the number of individuals at risk (denominator) (Agency for Healthcare Research and Quality, 2015). This method allows for the calculation of various types of key performance indicators (KPIs) in healthcare.

Proportion (%): This type of KPI measures the percentage of a specific outcome within a population. For example, the proportion of cardiovascular deaths that are male in the second quarter of a year.

Ratio (:): This KPI compares two related quantities. For instance, the ratio of male to female cardiovascular deaths in the third quarter of a year.

Count: This KPI simply counts the number of occurrences of a specific event, such as the number of tuberculosis cases in the first quarter of a year (Mainz, 2003).

Performance Measures and Performance Culture in Hospitals

Performance measures are essential for developing a performance culture within hospitals. These measures can be applied through various strategies:

1. **Leadership:** Strong leadership is crucial for fostering a culture of safety and quality. Leaders must be committed to patient safety and quality improvement, setting clear expectations and providing the necessary resources (The Joint Commission, 2023).
2. **Planning:** Effective planning involves setting measurable goals and developing strategies to achieve them. This includes identifying key

performance indicators (KPIs) and establishing benchmarks for quality and safety (Agency for Healthcare Research and Quality, 2015).

3. **Communication**: Open and transparent communication is vital for a performance culture. This includes regular reporting on performance metrics, sharing best practices, and encouraging feedback from staff and patients (The Joint Commission, 2023).

4. **Developing Staff Competencies**: Continuous education and training are essential for maintaining high standards of care. This involves providing ongoing professional development opportunities and ensuring that staff are competent in the latest best practices (World Health Organization, 2023).

5. **Continuous Employee Involvement**: Engaging employees in quality improvement initiatives helps to foster a sense of ownership and accountability. This can be achieved through regular team meetings, quality circles, and involving staff in decision-making processes (Agency for Healthcare Research and Quality, 2015).

6. **Education**: Education is a cornerstone of patient safety and quality improvement. This includes training healthcare professionals on safety protocols, quality improvement methodologies, and the importance of patient-centered care (World Health Organization, 2023).

7. **Implementation of an Open and Honest Reporting System**: Encouraging a culture of transparency where staff feel safe to report errors and near misses without fear of punishment is crucial. This helps to identify areas for improvement and prevent future incidents (The Joint Commission, 2023).

8. **Change to a Non-Punitive Culture**: Shifting from a blame culture to a learning culture where mistakes are seen as opportunities for improvement rather than reasons for punishment is essential for fostering a performance culture (Agency for Healthcare Research and Quality, 2015).

Communicating Standards in Healthcare

Effective communication of standards in healthcare is crucial for ensuring that all stakeholders understand and adhere to the established guidelines.

This process involves developing a comprehensive communication plan that addresses various aspects of communication.

Developing the Communication Plan

A communication plan is essential for systematically conveying standards to the intended audience. The plan should include the following components:

1. **Who is the Audience?** Identifying the target audience is the first step in developing a communication plan. The audience may include healthcare providers, administrative staff, patients, and other stakeholders (The Joint Commission, 2023).
2. **What Needs to Be Communicated?** Clearly defining the content that needs to be communicated is crucial. This includes the specific standards, guidelines, and any relevant updates or changes (World Health Organization, 2023).
3. **What Channels and Methods of Communication Will Be Used?** Selecting appropriate communication channels and methods is vital for effective dissemination. Options include employee handbooks, training workshops, formal conferences, newsletters, and informal talks (Agency for Healthcare Research and Quality, 2015).
4. **Who Will Be the Source of the Communication?** Identifying the source of the communication ensures that the information is credible and authoritative. This could be senior management, department heads, or designated communication officers (The Joint Commission, 2023).
5. **How Will the Communication Be Sequenced and Coordinated?** Planning the sequence and coordination of communication helps in delivering the message in a structured manner. This involves scheduling the communication activities and ensuring they are aligned with organizational goals (World Health Organization, 2023).
6. **How Will Feedback Be Obtained?** Establishing mechanisms for obtaining feedback is essential for assessing the effectiveness of the

communication. This can be done through surveys, feedback forms, and open forums (Agency for Healthcare Research and Quality, 2015).

7. **How Will the Communication Plan Be Evaluated?** Evaluating the communication plan involves assessing whether the standards reached the intended audience, were communicated without distortion, and were understood and applied correctly (The Joint Commission, 2023).

Methods for Communication

Various methods can be employed to communicate standards effectively:

- **Employee Handbooks/Manuals**
- **Training/Workshops**
- **Formal Conferences, Meetings, Seminars**
- **Supervision Programs**
- **Monitoring Programs**
- **Newsletters**
- **Informal Talks**
- **Job Aids** (World Health Organization, 2023)

Barriers to Communication

Effective communication can be hindered by various barriers, which can be categorized into sender and receiver barriers.

Sender Barriers:

- Use of unclear words, phrases, or terms.
- Distortion of standards due to deletions, additions, and changes.
- Communication at inappropriate times.
- Mismatch between the complexity of the information and the audience's understanding (Agency for Healthcare Research and Quality, 2015).

Receiver Barriers:

- Lack of understanding of the purpose of the standard.
- Belief that the standard will negatively impact their status.

- Perception that the standard was developed due to poor job performance.
- Requirement for cooperation among different groups (The Joint Commission, 2023).

Evaluation of the Communication Plan

Evaluating the communication plan involves several key questions:

- Did the standard reach the intended audience and individuals within those groups?
- Was the standard communicated without distortion?
- Was the standard communicated within the planned timeframe?
- Did the audience understand and apply the standard? (World Health Organization, 2023).

References:

1. Agency for Healthcare Research and Quality. (2015). Types of health care quality measures. Retrieved from https://www.ahrq.gov/talkingquality/measures/types.html
2. Agency for Healthcare Research and Quality. (2022). Quality Indicators (Qis). Retrieved from https://www.ahrq.gov/topics/quality-indicators-qis.html
3. American Academy of Family Physicians. (2023). Quality measures. Retrieved from https://www.aafp.org/family-physician/practice-and-career/managing-your-practice/quality-measures.html
4. American Medical Association. (2005). Performance-Improvement Continuing Medical Education (PI-CME). Retrieved from https://www.ama-assn.org
5. Cascade Strategy. (2023). 21 healthcare KPIs you should track (+ template). Retrieved from https://www.cascade.app/blog/healthcare-kpis
6. Centers for Disease Control and Prevention. (2023). Healthcare-associated Infections. Retrieved from https://www.cdc.gov/hai/index.html
7. Continu. (2023). Healthcare performance management: Definitive guide. Retrieved from https://www.continu.com/blog/performance-management-in-healthcare
8. Crosby, P. B. (1979). Quality is free: The art of making quality certain. McGraw-Hill.
9. Databox. (2023). 18 healthcare key performance indicators to include in a KPI dashboard. Retrieved from https://databox.com/healthcare-kpi-dashboard
10. Deming, W. E. (1986). Out of the crisis. MIT Press.
11. Donabedian, A. (1988). The quality of care: How can it be assessed? Journal of the American Medical Association, 260(12), 1743-1748. https://doi.org/10.1001/jama.1988.03410120089033
12. Health Information and Quality Authority (HIQA). (2013). Guidance on developing key performance indicators and minimum data sets to monitor healthcare quality. Dublin: Health Information and Quality Authority.
13. IBM. (2023). What are healthcare performance measurements? Retrieved from https://www.ibm.com/topics/healthcare-performance-measurements
14. Insightsoftware. (2024). 25 best healthcare KPIs and metric examples for 2024 reporting. Retrieved from https://insightsoftware.com/blog/25-best-healthcare-kpis-and-metric-examples/

15. Institute of Medicine. (1999). To err is human: Building a safer health system. National Academy Press.

16. Institute of Medicine. (2001). Crossing the quality chasm: A new health system for the 21st century. National Academy Press.

17. Joint Commission. (2023). Performance measurement. Retrieved from https://www.jointcommission.org/measurement/

18. Juran, J. M. (1988). Juran on planning for quality. Free Press.

19. KPI.org. (2023). How to develop KPIs / performance measures. Retrieved from https://www.kpi.org/KPI-Basics/KPI-Development/

20. Mainz, J. (2003). Defining and classifying clinical indicators for quality improvement. International Journal for Quality in Health Care, 15(6), 523-530. https://doi.org/10.1093/intqhc/mzg081

21. National Committee for Quality Assurance (NCQA). (1997). Healthcare Effectiveness Data and Information Set (HEDIS). Retrieved from https://www.ncqa.org

22. The Joint Commission. (2023). Patient safety. Retrieved from https://www.jointcommission.org/resources/patient-safety/

23. Wiley, M. M. (2015). The impact of electronic health records on healthcare quality. Journal of Health Information Management, 29(3), 45-52.

24. World Health Organization. (2023). Patient safety. Retrieved from https://www.who.int/news-room/fact-sheets/detail/patient-safety

Chapter 7

Patient Safety

Introduction and definition of patient safety:

Patient safety is a discipline that emphasizes safety in health care through the prevention, reduction, reporting, and analysis of medical error that often leads to adverse effects. According to the Institute of Medicine (IOM), patient safety is defined as "the prevention of harm to patients" and emphasizes the importance of creating systems that prevent errors and mitigate their effects when they occur (Kohn, Corrigan, & Donaldson, 2000). This definition highlights the proactive nature of patient safety efforts, focusing on preventing errors before they result in harm.

The World Health Organization (WHO) further elaborates that patient safety involves "the absence of preventable harm to a patient during the process of health care and the reduction of risk of unnecessary harm associated with health care to an acceptable minimum" (WHO, 2023). This definition underscores the dual goals of preventing harm and minimizing risks through systematic efforts.

Patient safety involves Reporting and **analysis** of medical errors. The Agency for Healthcare Research and Quality (AHRQ) emphasizes the importance of a culture of safety where healthcare professionals are encouraged to report errors and near misses without fear of retribution. This culture is essential for learning from mistakes and improving safety practices (AHRQ, 2019).

Evolution of the Science of Patient Safety

1950: Joint Commission on Accreditation of Hospitals (JCAHO)

The Joint Commission on Accreditation of Hospitals (JCAHO) was established in 1951 as an independent, not-for-profit organization in Chicago, Illinois. Its mission was to improve the quality of hospital care through the development of standards and the accreditation of hospitals (Joint Commission, n.d.).

1997: National Patient Safety Foundation (NPSF) Founded in the U.S.

The National Patient Safety Foundation (NPSF) was founded in 1997 to advance the safety of health care workers and patients. It aimed to disseminate strategies to prevent harm and improve patient safety through education, outreach, and research (National Patient Safety Foundation, 2017).

1999: To Err is Human

The landmark report "To Err is Human: Building a Safer Health System" was published by the Institute of Medicine in 1999. It revealed that between 44,000 and 98,000 people die annually in U.S. hospitals due to preventable medical errors, highlighting the urgent need for a comprehensive strategy to improve patient safety (Institute of Medicine, 1999).

2001: Crossing the Quality Chasm

In 2001, the Institute of Medicine released "Crossing the Quality Chasm: A New Health System for the 21st Century," which called for a fundamental redesign of the American health care system. The report identified six aims for improvement: safety, effectiveness, patient-centeredness, timeliness, efficiency, and equity (Institute of Medicine, 2001).

2003: The Joint Commission National Patient Safety Goals (NPSG)

The Joint Commission established the National Patient Safety Goals (NPSG) in 2002, with the first set becoming effective on January 1, 2003. These goals were designed to address specific areas of concern in patient safety and to improve the quality of care provided by accredited organizations (The Joint Commission, 2024).

2006: Joint Commission International (JCI) International Patient Safety Goals (IPSG)

In 2006, the Joint Commission International (JCI) developed the International Patient Safety Goals (IPSG) to help accredited organizations address critical areas of patient safety. These goals were adapted from the National Patient Safety Goals and have been monitored in JCI-accredited hospitals since their inception (Joint Commission International, 2020).

2007: Lucian Leape Institute for Patient Safety

The Lucian Leape Institute was established in 2007 by the National Patient Safety Foundation to provide a strategic vision for improving patient safety. Named after Dr. Lucian Leape, the institute functions as a think tank to identify new approaches and innovations necessary for significant improvements in patient safety (Institute for Healthcare Improvement, 2023).

2017: NPSF and IHI Merge

In May 2017, the National Patient Safety Foundation (NPSF) merged with the Institute for Healthcare Improvement (IHI) to combine their efforts in advancing patient safety. This merger aimed to create a unified organization with a stronger focus on improving patient safety and health care quality (Institute for Healthcare Improvement, 2017).

2021: Global Patient Safety Action Plan (GPSAP) 2021–2030

The World Health Organization (WHO) adopted the Global Patient Safety Action Plan (GPSAP) 2021–2030 in 2021. This plan aims to implement policies, programs, and strategic interventions to improve patient safety globally. Progress has been made, although some core indicators still require attention (World Health Organization, 2024).

2022: Significant National Patient Safety Improvement

A study published in JAMA in 2022, funded by the Agency for Healthcare Research and Quality (AHRQ), showed significant reductions in in-hospital adverse events in the U.S. from 2010 to 2019. The study highlighted improvements in patient safety for conditions such as heart attack, heart failure, pneumonia, and major surgeries (Agency for Healthcare Research and Quality, 2022).

2024: Updated National Patient Safety Goals

The Joint Commission continues to update its National Patient Safety Goals annually. The 2024 goals focus on significant problems in health care safety and specific actions to prevent them, including suicide prevention, reducing harm from anticoagulant therapy, and improving communication among caregivers (The Joint Commission, 2024).

Swiss Cheese Model

The Swiss Cheese Model, developed by James Reason, is a metaphor used to illustrate how errors occur in complex systems. It likens human systems to multiple slices of Swiss cheese, each with holes representing potential failures. When these holes align, they create a pathway for errors to manifest, leading to adverse events (Reason, 1990).

Why do errors happen?

James Reason proposes that errors occur due to two main types of failures:

1. **Execution Error**: The intended action is wrong.
2. **Planning Error**: The action did not go as intended.

Additionally, Reason distinguishes between two types of errors:

1. **Active Errors (Sharp End)**: These occur at the level of the frontline operator and their effects are felt almost immediately. Examples include a nurse administering the wrong medication or a pilot making a navigation error (Reason, 1990).

2. **Latent Errors (Blunt End)**: These are hidden problems within the system, such as poor design, incorrect installation, faulty maintenance, bad management decisions, and poorly structured organizations. These errors may lie dormant for a long time until they contribute to an adverse event (Reason, 1990).

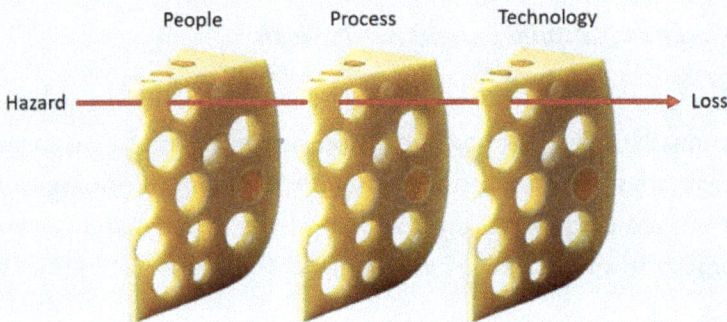

Figure 7.1: Swiss cheese model

Types of Medical Errors:

In patient safety, understanding the various types of errors and adverse events is crucial for improving healthcare quality and patient outcomes. Here are detailed descriptions of these types, along with examples and additional relevant types:

1. **Adverse Events**: These are injuries caused by medical management rather than the underlying condition of the patient. They can be preventable or non-preventable.

   o **Example 1**: A patient develops a severe infection after surgery due to improper sterilization of surgical instruments (preventable).

- Example 2: A patient experiences an allergic reaction to a medication despite no known allergies (non-preventable) (Agency for Healthcare Research and Quality [AHRQ], 2019).

2. **Errors**: Errors are acts of commission (doing something wrong) or omission (failing to do the right thing) that lead to an undesirable outcome or a significant potential for such an outcome.

- Example 1: Administering the wrong dosage of medication to a patient (commission).
- Example 2: Failing to administer a necessary medication (omission) (Reason, 1990).

3. **Slips and Lapses**: These are failures in the execution of an action, often due to attention or memory failures. Slips are observable actions, while lapses are internal events.

- Slip Example 1: A nurse accidentally administers medication to the wrong patient due to a momentary lapse in attention.
- Slip Example 2: A surgeon inadvertently cuts the wrong tissue during an operation.
- Lapse Example 1: A doctor forgets to document a patient's allergy in their medical record.
- Lapse Example 2: A nurse forgets to administer a scheduled dose of medication (Reason, 1990).

4. **Medication Errors**: These involve any preventable event that may cause or lead to inappropriate medication use or patient harm while the medication is in the control of the healthcare professional, patient, or consumer.

- Example 1: Prescribing a medication that the patient is allergic to.
- Example 2: Dispensing the wrong medication due to a labeling error (World Health Organization [WHO], 2023).

5. **Sentinel Events**: These are unexpected occurrences involving death or serious physical or psychological injury, or the risk thereof. Types of sentinel events include:

   o **Example 1**: Patient suicide while under care.
   o **Example 2: Assault/Rape/Sexual Assault of a Patient**.
   o **Example 3: Patient Elopement** is When a patient who is cognitively, physically, mentally, emotionally, or chemically impaired wanders away, walks away, runs away, escapes, or otherwise leaves the healthcare facility unsupervised, unnoticed, and/or prior to their scheduled discharge.
   o **Example 4: Fire**, any instance of fire within the healthcare facility that leads to patient harm.
   o **Example 5: Infant Abduction**, unauthorized removal of an infant from the healthcare facility.
   o **Example 6: Infant Discharge to the Wrong Family**.
   o **Example 7:** Severe Maternal Morbidity and Mortality, which are severe complications during childbirth that result in significant maternal injury or death.
   o **Example 8: Severe Neonatal Hyperbilirubinemia**, which is excessive bilirubin levels in a newborn that can lead to serious complications.
   o **Example 9: Prolonged Fluoroscopy with Cumulative Dose over 1500 rads to a Single Field** Excessive radiation exposure during medical imaging procedures.
   o **Example 10: Radiation Overdose,** which is administration of radiation doses that exceed the prescribed amount.
   o **Example 11:** Unintended Retention of a Foreign Object, when objects are left inside a patient after surgery.
   o **Example 12: Wrong Patient, Wrong Site, Wrong Procedure** (The Joint Commission, 2023).

6. **Preventable and Non-Preventable Errors**:

   o **Preventable Errors**: These are errors that could have been avoided with the application of accepted standards of care.

- Example 1: A patient develops a pressure ulcer due to inadequate turning and repositioning.
- Example 2: A patient receives the wrong blood type during a transfusion due to a labeling error.

o **Non-Preventable Errors**: These occur despite the application of accepted standards of care and are often due to the inherent risks of medical treatment.

- Example 1: A patient experiences an adverse reaction to a medication despite proper administration and monitoring.
- Example 2: A patient develops a post-operative infection despite adherence to sterile techniques (AHRQ, 2019).

7. **Near Misses**: These are incidents that could have resulted in harm but did not, either by chance or through timely intervention.

o **Example 1**: A nurse catches a medication error before administering the drug to the patient.

o **Example 2**: A surgeon realizes a mistake in the surgical plan before making an incision (AHRQ, 2019).

8. **Diagnostic Errors**: These occur when there is a failure to establish an accurate and timely explanation of the patient's health problem(s) or a failure to communicate that explanation to the patient.

o **Example 1**: A patient is misdiagnosed with a viral infection when they actually have bacterial meningitis.

o **Example 2**: A delay in diagnosing a patient with cancer, leading to progression of the disease (Singh et al., 2017).

9. **Surgical Errors**: These include wrong-site surgery, retained surgical instruments, and other mistakes that occur during surgical procedures.

o **Example 1**: Performing surgery on the wrong limb.

o **Example 2**: Leaving a surgical sponge inside a patient (Gawande et al., 1999).

10. **Healthcare-Associated Infections (HAIs)**: These are infections that patients acquire while receiving treatment for other conditions within a healthcare setting.

   o **Example 1**: A patient develops a catheter-associated urinary tract infection.
   o **Example 2**: A patient contracts a surgical site infection after an operation (Magill et al., 2014).

11. **Patient Falls**: Falls are common adverse events in hospitals, particularly among elderly patients.

   o **Example 1**: An elderly patient falls while trying to get out of bed without assistance.
   o **Example 2**: A patient slips in the bathroom due to a wet floor (Oliver et al., 2007).

12. **Pressure Ulcers**: Also known as bedsores, these are injuries to the skin and underlying tissue resulting from prolonged pressure on the skin.

   o **Example 1**: A patient develops a pressure ulcer on their heel due to prolonged immobility.
   o **Example 2**: A patient develops a pressure ulcer on their sacrum due to inadequate repositioning (National Pressure Injury Advisory Panel, 2016).

13. **Unsafe Blood Transfusions**: Errors in blood transfusion practices can lead to serious adverse reactions and infections.

   o **Example 1**: A patient receives the wrong blood type due to a labeling error.
   o **Example 2**: A patient contracts an infection from improperly screened blood (WHO, 2023).

14. **Patient Misidentification**: This occurs when patients are incorrectly identified, leading to errors such as wrong-site surgery or incorrect medication administration.

   o **Example 1**: A patient receives another patient's medication due to a mix-up in identification.

o **Example 2**: A patient undergoes a procedure intended for another patient (The Joint Commission, 2023).

15. **Unsafe Injection Practices**: These include the reuse of needles or syringes and improper handling of injection equipment, which can lead to infections and other complications.

o **Example 1**: Reusing a syringe for multiple patients, leading to the spread of infections.
o **Example 2**: Using non-sterile needles, resulting in patient infections (WHO, 2023).

IOM reports and patient safety

The reports "To Err is Human" and "Crossing the Quality Chasm" by the Institute of Medicine (IOM) have been pivotal in revolutionizing patient safety awareness and healthcare quality.

To Err is Human

The "To Err is Human" report, published in 2000, brought to light the alarming prevalence of medical errors in the United States. It revealed that adverse events occurred in 2.9% of hospitalizations in New York and 3.7% in Colorado and Utah. Of these adverse events, 13.6% resulted in deaths in New York, and 6.6% in Colorado and Utah (IOM, 2000). The report estimated that at least 44,000 and up to 98,000 deaths occur annually in the U.S. due to medical errors (IOM, 2000). This staggering statistic highlighted the urgent need for systemic changes in healthcare to improve patient safety.

Globally, the impact of medical errors is also significant. The World Health Organization (WHO) reports that around 1 in every 10 patients is harmed in healthcare, with more than 3 million deaths occurring annually due to unsafe care. In low-to-middle-income countries, as many as 4 in 100 people die from unsafe care (WHO, 2023). These figures underscore the universal challenge of patient safety and the necessity for global efforts to address it.

Crossing the Quality Chasm

Following the "To Err is Human" report, the IOM published "Crossing the Quality Chasm: A New Health System for the 21st Century" in 2001. This report outlined a comprehensive framework for improving healthcare quality, emphasizing six key aims:

- **Safety**: Avoiding harm to patients from the care that is intended to help them.
- **Timeliness**: Reducing waits and sometimes harmful delays for both those who receive and those who give care.
- **Effectiveness**: Providing services based on scientific knowledge to all who could benefit and refraining from providing services to those not likely to benefit.
- **Efficiency**: Avoiding waste, including waste of equipment, supplies, ideas, and energy.
- **Equity**: Providing care that does not vary in quality because of personal characteristics such as gender, ethnicity, geographic location, and socioeconomic status.
- **Personalized Care**: Ensuring that patient values guide all clinical decisions (IOM, 2001).

These reports collectively shifted the focus of healthcare from individual blame to systemic improvement. They emphasized the need for a culture of safety, continuous quality improvement, and patient-centered care. The recommendations from these reports have led to the development of numerous safety protocols, quality improvement initiatives, and regulatory changes that continue to shape healthcare practices today.

Medical Errors in Canada

In Canada, there was an adverse event rate of 7.5 per 100 hospital admissions from the 3,745 charts that were studied. For the 2.5 million annual hospital admissions in Canada, this translates to about 185,000 adverse events, of which just under 70,000 could be classified as medical errors, the report stated (Baker et al., 2004).

Also in Canada, annual deaths from adverse events were calculated to be between 9,250 and 23,750 (Baker et al., 2004).

More statistics on medical errors from Johns Hopkins

In 2016, analyzing medical death rate data over an eight-year period, Johns Hopkins patient safety experts calculated that more than 250,000 deaths per year are due to medical error in the U.S. This figure indicates that 10 percent of all U.S. deaths are now due to medical error, making it the third highest cause of death in the U.S., after heart disease and cancer (Makary & Daniel, 2016). The study highlighted that medical errors are an under-recognized cause of death (Makary & Daniel, 2016).

More statistics on medical errors reveal that roughly 10 percent of U.S. deaths annually are due to system-wide failings and poorly coordinated care. Preventable medical errors cost the country tens of billions of dollars each year (Institute of Medicine, 2000). Additionally, one in three patients admitted to the hospital will experience a medical error or preventable harm (James, 2013). Studies of wrong-site, wrong-surgery, and wrong-patient procedures show that "never events" are happening at an alarming rate of up to 40 times per week in U.S. hospitals (Seiden & Barach, 2006).

Makary and Daniel (2016) called for reforms to improve the reporting of medical errors, which could inform prevention efforts. In a letter dated May 1, 2016, they asked the Centers for Disease Control and Prevention (CDC) to rank medical errors on the list of leading causes of death and to alter death certificates so that medical errors contributing to a patient's death can be routinely reported by doctors, medical examiners, and coroners.

European Data from WHO

Medical errors and health-care related adverse events occur in 8% to 12% of hospitalizations. The United Kingdom Department of Health estimated about 850,000 adverse events a year, which is approximately 10%

of hospital admissions. Spain, in its 2005 national study of adverse events, and France and Denmark have published incidence studies with similar results (World Health Organization [WHO], 2023).

European Infection Rate in Hospitals

Infections associated with health care affect an estimated 1 in 20 hospital patients on average every year, which is estimated at 4.1 million patients. The four most common types of infections are urinary tract infections (27%), lower respiratory tract infections (24%), surgical site infections (17%), and bloodstream infections (10.5%). Multiresistant Staphylococcus aureus (MRSA) is isolated in about 5% of all infections associated with health care. The United Kingdom National Audit Office estimates the cost of such infections at £1 billion per year (European Centre for Disease Prevention and Control [ECDC], 2024).

More EU Stats on Medical Errors

While 23% of European Union citizens claim to have been directly affected by medical error, 18% claim to have experienced a serious medical error in a hospital, and 11% to have been prescribed the wrong medication. Evidence on medical errors shows that 50% to 70.2% of such harm can be prevented through comprehensive systematic approaches to patient safety. Statistics show that strategies to reduce the rate of adverse events in the European Union alone would lead to the prevention of more than 750,000 harm-inflicting medical errors per year, leading in turn to over 3.2 million fewer days of hospitalization, 260,000 fewer incidents of permanent disability, and 95,000 fewer deaths per year (WHO, 2023).

WHO 10 Facts on Patient Safety

Patient safety is a serious global public health issue. Estimates show that in developed countries as many as one in 10 patients is harmed while receiving hospital care. Of every 100 hospitalized patients at any given time, seven in developed and 10 in developing countries will acquire health care-associated infections. Hundreds of millions of patients are affected by this worldwide each year (WHO, 2023).

Serious Medical Missteps

The main kinds of serious medical mistakes, as reported by 114 interns and residents who responded anonymously to a questionnaire about their own most significant errors in the last year, include the following categories:

1. **Diagnostic Errors**: These occur when there is a failure to establish an accurate and timely explanation of the patient's health problem(s) or a failure to communicate that explanation to the patient.

   o **Example 1**: Misdiagnosing a heart attack as indigestion.
   o **Example 2**: Delayed diagnosis of cancer, leading to progression of the disease (Makary & Daniel, 2016).

2. **Medication Errors**: These involve any preventable event that may cause or lead to inappropriate medication use or patient harm while the medication is in the control of the healthcare professional, patient, or consumer.

   o **Example 1**: Administering the wrong dosage of a medication.
   o **Example 2**: Prescribing a medication that the patient is allergic to (Makary & Daniel, 2016).

3. **Surgical Errors**: These include wrong-site surgery, retained surgical instruments, and other mistakes that occur during surgical procedures.

   o **Example 1**: Performing surgery on the wrong limb.
   o **Example 2**: Leaving a surgical sponge inside a patient after an operation (Seiden & Barach, 2006).

4. **Infections**: These are healthcare-associated infections that patients acquire while receiving treatment for other conditions within a healthcare setting.

   o **Example 1**: A patient develops a catheter-associated urinary tract infection.

o   **Example 2**: A patient contracts a surgical site infection after an operation (ECDC, 2024).

5. **Falls**: These are common adverse events in hospitals, particularly among elderly patients.

o   **Example 1**: An elderly patient falls while trying to get out of bed without assistance.

o   **Example 2**: A patient slips in the bathroom due to a wet floor (Oliver et al., 2007).

6. **Pressure Ulcers**: Also known as bedsores, these are injuries to the skin and underlying tissue resulting from prolonged pressure on the skin.

o   **Example 1**: A patient develops a pressure ulcer on their heel due to prolonged immobility.

o   **Example 2**: A patient develops a pressure ulcer on their sacrum due to inadequate repositioning (National Pressure Injury Advisory Panel, 2016).

People Are Set-Up to Make Mistakes

Incompetent people are, at most, 1% of the problem. The other 99% are good people trying to do a good job who make very simple mistakes, and it's the processes that set them up to make these mistakes (Leape, 2005).

Dr. Lucian Leape from the Harvard School of Public Health emphasizes that "the transforming insight for medicine from human factors research is that errors are rarely due to personal failing, inadequacies, and carelessness. Rather, they result from defects in the design and conditions of medical work that lead careful, competent, caring physicians and nurses to make mistakes that are often no different from the simple mistakes people make every day, but which have devastating consequences for patients. Errors result from faulty systems, not from faulty people, so it is the systems that must be fixed. Errors are excusable; ignoring them is not" (Leape, 2005).

A Just Culture:

A just culture Is one that supports the discussion of errors so that lessons can be learned from them. James Reason, a prominent figure in the field of human factors and safety, emphasized that a just culture is essential for improving safety in healthcare. He stated, "The transforming insight for medicine from human factors research is that errors are rarely due to personal failing, inadequacies, and carelessness. Rather, they result from defects in the design and conditions of medical work that lead careful, competent, caring physicians and nurses to make mistakes that are often no different from the simple mistakes people make every day, but which have devastating consequences for patients. Errors result from faulty systems, not from faulty people, so it is the systems that must be fixed. Errors are excusable; ignoring them is not" (Leape, 2005).

Need to Increase Focus on the Human Factors:

Studies of adverse patient incidents have heightened our awareness of the need to redesign processes to prevent human errors. Human factors research has shown that many errors in healthcare are not due to individual negligence but are the result of systemic issues. This understanding has led to the recognition that improving patient safety requires a focus on the design of healthcare systems and processes.

It Is time for organizations to use cognitive ergonomics or human factors analysis to make healthcare services safer for patients.

Cognitive ergonomics involves understanding how cognitive processes such as perception, memory, and reasoning affect interactions with other elements of a system. By applying principles of human factors, healthcare organizations can design systems that support the cognitive abilities of healthcare providers, reduce the likelihood of errors, and enhance overall patient safety (Carayon et al., 2006).

National Patient Safety Goals (NPSG)

The Joint Commission implemented the National Patient Safety Goals (NPSG) in 2002, with the first set of guidelines officially introduced on

January 1, 2003 (Wolters Kluwer, 2024). The primary aim of these goals was to address specific areas of concern regarding patient safety and to provide a framework for healthcare organizations to improve safety practices (PSNet, 2024). The NPSGs were developed based on input from practitioners, provider organizations, purchasers, consumer groups, and other stakeholders (Joint Commission, 2024).

As of 2024, the NPSGs include several key standards designed to enhance patient safety across various healthcare settings. These standards focus on critical areas such as patient identification, communication among caregivers, medication safety, clinical alarm safety, infection prevention, fall prevention, pressure ulcer prevention, risk assessment, and health care equity (Joint Commission, 2024). The specific goals are:

1. Improve the accuracy of patient identification.
2. Improve the effectiveness of communication among caregivers.
3. Improve the safety of using medications.
4. Reduce patient harm associated with clinical alarm systems.
5. Reduce the risk of health care-associated infections.
6. Reduce the risk of patient harm resulting from falls.
7. Prevent health care-associated pressure ulcers.
8. Identify safety risks inherent in the patient population.
9. Improve health care equity (Joint Commission, 2024).

International Patient Safety Goals (IPSG)

The Joint Commission International (JCI) implemented the International Patient Safety Goals (IPSG) in 2006. These goals were adapted from the Joint Commission's National Patient Safety Goals to address specific patient safety concerns in the international context (Joint Commission International, 2024). The IPSGs aim to promote specific improvements in patient safety by focusing on six key areas identified as problematic in healthcare settings (Joint Commission International, 2024).

The current IPSG standards are:

1. Identify patients correctly.
2. Improve effective communication.

3. Improve the safety of high-alert medications.
4. Ensure safe surgery.
5. Reduce the risk of health care-associated infections.
6. Reduce the risk of patient harm resulting from falls (Joint Commission International, 2024).

Essential Safety Requirements (ESR) by CBAHI

The Saudi Central Board for Accreditation of Healthcare Institutions (CBAHI) implemented the Essential Safety Requirements (ESR) to ensure patient safety and protection against healthcare-related errors. The ESR standards were introduced as a mandatory set of conditions that hospitals must comply with to receive national accreditation from CBAHI (CBAHI, 2024).

The current ESR standards include 20 national standards that cover various aspects of patient safety. These standards address areas such as the verification of credentials, privileging processes, safety in handling and administration of blood products, VTE screening and management, correct patient identification, surgical safety checklists, anesthesiologist qualifications, staff training for moderate sedation, infection control, negative pressure isolation room adequacy, handling high-alert medications, medication error reporting, disease transmission prevention, fire safety, radiation safety, and medical gas system maintenance (CBAHI, 2024). The 20 ESR standards are:

1. Proper credentialing of staff members licensed to provide patient care.
2. Medical staff members have current delineated clinical privileges.
3. Policies and procedures guide the handling, use, and administration of blood and blood products.
4. Patients at risk for developing venous thromboembolism are identified and managed.
5. The hospital has a process to ensure correct identification of patients.
6. The hospital has a process to prevent wrong patient, wrong site, and wrong surgery/procedure.
7. Anesthesia staff members have the appropriate qualifications.

8. Staff training for moderate sedation.
9. Infection control practices.
10. Adequacy of negative pressure isolation rooms.
11. Handling of high-alert medications.
12. Medication error reporting system.
13. Disease transmission prevention.
14. Fire safety measures.
15. Radiation safety protocols.
16. Maintenance of medical gas systems.
17. Patient safety risk assessment.
18. Implementation of surgical safety checklists.
19. Monitoring and reporting of transfusion reactions.
20. Ensuring safe administration of blood transfusions (CBAHI, 2024).

Root Cause Analysis (RCA)

Root Cause Analysis (RCA) is a systematic process used to identify the underlying causes of problems or adverse events in healthcare settings. It aims to prevent recurrence by addressing the root causes rather than just the symptoms (Institute for Healthcare Improvement, 2023).

When to Start an RCA in a Hospital

An RCA should be initiated in a hospital setting when a significant adverse event occurs, such as a sentinel event, which is an unexpected occurrence involving death or serious physical or psychological injury (VHA National Center for Patient Safety, 2020). Additionally, RCAs can be conducted for near misses or any event that could have led to harm but did not, either by chance or timely intervention (Agency for Healthcare Research and Quality, 2023).

RCA on the Washington Monument

The RCA conducted on the Washington Monument is a classic example often cited to illustrate the process. The monument was deteriorating due to frequent cleaning with harsh chemicals. The RCA revealed that the cleaning was necessary because of excessive bird droppings, which were due to a large population of spiders. The spiders were there because of an abundance of insects attracted by the monument's lighting at dusk. The solution was to change the lighting schedule to reduce the insect population, thereby reducing the spiders and bird droppings (Sologic, 2020).

Steps of RCA in Healthcare

The RCA process in healthcare typically involves the following steps:

1. **Charter a Team**: Assemble a multidisciplinary team with the necessary expertise.
2. **Define the Problem**: Clearly describe the adverse event or issue.
3. **Collect Data**: Gather detailed information about the event, including timelines, personnel involved, and environmental conditions.
4. **Identify Root Causes**: Use tools like the "5 Whys" or fishbone diagrams to drill down to the underlying causes.
5. **Develop Action Plan**: Create strategies to address the root causes and prevent recurrence.
6. **Implement Solutions**: Put the action plan into practice.
7. **Evaluate Effectiveness**: Monitor the outcomes to ensure the solutions are effective (VHA National Center for Patient Safety, 2020).

Example of RCA in Healthcare

An example of RCA in healthcare involved a hospital that experienced a series of medication errors. The RCA team discovered that the errors were due to similar packaging of different medications, leading to confusion among staff. The action plan included redesigning the packaging to make it more distinct and implementing additional checks during medication administration. As a result, the hospital saw a significant reduction in medication errors, improving patient safety and care quality (Institute for Healthcare Improvement, 2023).

Failure Modes and Effects Analysis (FMEA)

Failure Modes and Effects Analysis (FMEA) is a systematic, proactive method for evaluating a process to identify where and how it might fail and to assess the relative impact of different failures in order to identify the parts of the process that are most in need of change (Institute for Healthcare Improvement, 2024).

When is FMEA Used in Healthcare?

FMEA is used in healthcare to anticipate and prevent potential failures before they occur. It is particularly useful in evaluating new processes prior to implementation and in assessing the impact of proposed changes to existing processes (Agency for Healthcare Research and Quality, 2023). Common applications include medication management, patient handoffs, and surgical procedures (Institute for Healthcare Improvement, 2024).

Steps to Perform FMEA

1. **Select a Process to Analyze**: Choose a process that is known to be problematic or has the potential for significant impact if it fails (Institute for Healthcare Improvement, 2024).
2. **Assemble a Cross-Functional Team**: Form a multidisciplinary team that includes members with different perspectives and expertise related to the process (Quality-One, 2024).
3. **Describe the Process**: Create a detailed flowchart of the process to be analyzed, ensuring all team members understand each step (VHA National Center for Patient Safety, 2020).
4. **Identify Failure Modes**: For each step in the process, identify all the ways in which it could fail (Institute for Healthcare Improvement, 2024).
5. **Determine the Effects of Each Failure**: Assess the potential consequences of each failure mode (Quality-One, 2024).
6. **Assign Severity, Occurrence, and Detection Ratings**: Rate each failure mode based on its severity, the likelihood of occurrence, and the likelihood of detection before it causes harm (VHA National Center for Patient Safety, 2020).

7. **Calculate the Risk Priority Number (RPN)**: Multiply the severity, occurrence, and detection ratings to prioritize the failure modes (Institute for Healthcare Improvement, 2024).

8. **Develop Action Plans**: Create strategies to reduce or eliminate the high-priority failure modes (Quality-One, 2024).

9. **Implement and Monitor the Action Plans**: Put the action plans into practice and monitor their effectiveness over time (VHA National Center for Patient Safety, 2020).

Calculating the Risk Priority Number (RPN)

RPN Calculation Formula:
RPN = Severity (S) × Occurrence (O) × Detection (D)

Scoring Criteria:

Severity (S) Scale (1-10):

1-3: Minor impact on patient
4-6: Moderate patient impact
7-10: Severe patient harm potential

Occurrence (O) Scale (1-10):

1-3: Rare occurrence
4-6: Occasional occurrence
7-10: Frequent occurrence

Detection (D) Scale (1-10):

1-3: High probability of detection
4-6: Moderate detection capability
7-10: Low probability of detection

Simplified Healthcare Example:

Medication Administration Error

- Severity: Incorrect medication dosage (potential for patient harm) = 8

- Occurrence: Frequency of medication administration errors = 6
- Detection: Likelihood of catching error before patient harm = 4

RPN Calculation:
RPN = $8 \times 6 \times 4 = 192$ (Carroll, 2009)

Example of a Successful FMEA in U.S. Hospitals

A notable example of a successful FMEA implementation in a U.S. hospital involved the administration of unfractionated heparin at a 367-bed academic pediatric hospital. The FMEA identified 233 potential points of failure, including mathematical errors, unknown requirements for administration, incorrect timing, difficulties accessing information from the hospital's electronic medical records (EMR), poor patient education, and the potential to administer incorrect dosages (Proactive Perioperative Risk Analysis, 2020).

The hospital implemented several countermeasures, such as standardizing heparin dosing protocols, improving EMR access, and enhancing staff training. These actions led to a statistically significant improvement in safety scores and a reduction in medication errors. The benefits included improved patient safety, enhanced staff confidence, and better compliance with medication administration protocols. However, challenges included the time and resources required to conduct the FMEA and implement the changes, as well as the need for ongoing monitoring and adjustment of the new processes (Proactive Perioperative Risk Analysis, 2020).

References:

1. Agency for Healthcare Research and Quality. (2019). Adverse Events, Near Misses, and Errors. Retrieved from https://psnet.ahrq.gov/primer/adverse-events-near-misses-and-errors

2. Agency for Healthcare Research and Quality. (2019). Patient Safety Network. Retrieved from https://psnet.ahrq.gov/

3. Agency for Healthcare Research and Quality. (2022). Major Study Finds Significant National Patient Safety Improvement. Retrieved from https://www.ahrq.gov/news/newsroom/press-releases/significant-patient-safety-improvement.html

4. Agency for Healthcare Research and Quality. (2023). Strategies and approaches for investigating patient safety events. Retrieved from https://psnet.ahrq.gov/primer/strategies-and-approaches-investigating-patient-safety-events

5. Baker, G. R., Norton, P. G., Flintoft, V., Blais, R., Brown, A., Cox, J., ... & Tamblyn, R. (2004). The Canadian Adverse Events Study: the incidence of adverse events among hospital patients in Canada. CMAJ, 170(11), 1678-1686. https://doi.org/10.1503/cmaj.1040918

6. CBAHI. (2024). Essential National Requirements for Patient Safety. Retrieved from https://portal.cbahi.gov.sa/english/patient-safety/essential-safety-requirements

7. Carroll, R. (2009). Risk management handbook for healthcare organizations. Jossey-Bass.

8. Carayon, P., Schoofs Hundt, A., Karsh, B. T., Gurses, A. P., Alvarado, C. J., Smith, M., & Flatley Brennan, P. (2006). Work system design for patient safety: the SEIPS model. Quality and Safety in Health Care, 15(Suppl 1), i50-i58. https://doi.org/10.1136/qshc.2005.015842

9. European Centre for Disease Prevention and Control. (2024). Point prevalence survey of healthcare-associated infections and antimicrobial use in European acute care hospitals 2022-2023. Retrieved from https://www.ecdc.europa.eu/en/publications-data/PPS-HAI-AMR-acute-care-europe-2022-2023

10. Gawande, A. A., Thomas, E. J., Zinner, M. J., & Brennan, T. A. (1999). The incidence and nature of surgical adverse events in Colorado and Utah in 1992. Surgery, 126(1), 66-75.

11. Institute for Healthcare Improvement. (2017). National Patient Safety Foundation and Institute for Healthcare Improvement to merge in May.

Modern Healthcare. Retrieved from
https://www.modernhealthcare.com/article/20170313/NEWS/17031999
1/national-patient-safety-foundation-and-institute-for-healthcare-
improvement-to-merge-in-may

12. Institute for Healthcare Improvement. (2023). IHI Lucian Leape Institute.
Retrieved from https://www.ihi.org/networks/initiatives/ihi-lucian-leape-
institute

13. Institute for Healthcare Improvement. (2023). RCA2: Improving root cause
analyses and actions to prevent harm. Retrieved from
https://www.ihi.org/resources/tools/rca2-improving-root-cause-analyses-
and-actions-prevent-harm

14. Institute for Healthcare Improvement. (2024). Failure Modes and Effects
Analysis (FMEA). Retrieved from
https://www.ihi.org/sites/default/files/SafetyToolkit_
FailureModesandEffectsAnalysis.pdf

15. Institute of Medicine. (1999). To Err is Human: Building a Safer Health
System. National Academies Press. Retrieved from
https://nap.nationalacademies.org/resource/9728/To-Err-is-Human-1999-
report-brief.pdf

16. Institute of Medicine. (2000). To Err is Human: Building a Safer Health
System. Washington, DC: National Academies Press.

17. Institute of Medicine. (2001). Crossing the Quality Chasm: A New Health
System for the 21st Century. National Academies Press. Retrieved from
https://www.ihi.org/resources/publications/crossing-quality-chasm-new-
health-system-21st-century

18. James, J. T. (2013). A new, evidence-based estimate of patient harms
associated with hospital care. Journal of Patient Safety, 9(3), 122-128.
https://doi.org/10.1097/PTS.0b013e3182948a69

19. Joint Commission. (n.d.). History of The Joint Commission. Retrieved from
https://www.jointcommission.org/who-we-are/facts-about-the-joint-
commission/history-of-the-joint-commission/

20. Joint Commission. (2024). National Patient Safety Goals. Retrieved from
https://www.jointcommission.org/standards/national-patient-safety-goals/

21. Joint Commission International. (2020). International Patient Safety Goals.
Retrieved from
https://www.jointcommissioninternational.org/standards/international-
patient-safety-goals/

22. Joint Commission International. (2024). International Patient Safety Goals. Retrieved from https://www.jointcommissioninternational.org/standards/international-patient-safety-goals/

23. Leape, L. L. (2005). IOM Medical Error Figures Are Not Exaggerated. JAMA, 293(19), 2384-2390. https://doi.org/10.1001/jama.293.19.2384

24. Magill, S. S., Edwards, J. R., Bamberg, W., Beldavs, Z. G., Dumyati, G., Kainer, M. A., ... & Fridkin, S. K. (2014). Multistate point-prevalence survey of health care–associated infections. New England Journal of Medicine, 370(13), 1198-1208.

25. Makary, M. A., & Daniel, M. (2016). Medical error—the third leading cause of death in the US. BMJ, 353, i2139. https://doi.org/10.1136/bmj.i2139

26. National Patient Safety Foundation. (2017). National Patient Safety Foundation. Retrieved from https://www.npsf.org/page/aboutus

27. National Pressure Injury Advisory Panel. (2016). Prevention and Treatment of Pressure Ulcers/Injuries: Clinical Practice Guideline. Retrieved from https://npiap.com/

28. Oliver, D., Healey, F., & Haines, T. P. (2007). Preventing falls and fall-related injuries in hospitals. Clinics in Geriatric Medicine, 23(4), 645-667.

29. Proactive Perioperative Risk Analysis. (2020). Use of Failure Mode and Effects Analysis (FMEA) in healthcare. Retrieved from https://www.apsf.org/article/proactive-perioperative-risk-analysis-use-of-failure-mode-and-effects-analysis-fmea/

30. PSNet. (2024). National Patient Safety Goals. Retrieved from https://psnet.ahrq.gov/primer/national-patient-safety-goals

31. Quality-One. (2024). Healthcare FMEA | Healthcare Failure Mode & Effects Analysis. Retrieved from https://quality-one.com/hfmea/

32. Reason, J. (1990). Human Error. Cambridge University Press.

33. Reason, J. (2000). Human error: models and management. BMJ, 320(7237), 768-770. Retrieved from https://www.bmj.com/content/320/7237/768

34. Seiden, A. M., & Barach, P. (2006). Wrong-side/wrong-site, wrong-procedure, and wrong-patient adverse events: Are they preventable? Archives of Surgery, 141(9), 931-939. https://doi.org/10.1001/archsurg.141.9.931

35. Singh, H., Schiff, G. D., Graber, M. L., Onakpoya, I., & Thompson, M. J. (2017). The global burden of diagnostic errors in primary care. BMJ Quality & Safety, 26(6), 484-494.

36. Sologic. (2020). 5 Whys and the monumental mystery. Retrieved from https://www.sologic.com/en-gb/resources/blog/english-uk/5-whys-and-the-monumental-mystery

37. The Joint Commission. (2023). Sentinel Event Policy and Procedures. Retrieved from https://www.jointcommission.org/resources/patient-safety-topics/sentinel-event/

38. VHA National Center for Patient Safety. (2020). Guide to performing a root cause analysis. Retrieved from https://www.patientsafety.va.gov/docs/RCA_Guidebook_10212020.pdf

39. Wolters Kluwer. (2024). National patient safety goals for hospitals. Retrieved from https://www.wolterskluwer.com/en/expert-insights/national-patient-safety-goals-for-hospitals

40. World Health Organization. (2023). Patient safety. Retrieved from https://www.who.int/news-room/fact-sheets/detail/patient-safety

41. World Health Organization. (2024). Progress on patient safety on track. Retrieved from https://www.who.int/news/item/18-06-2024-progress-on-patient-safety-on-track

Chapter 8

Quality Tools

This chapter will cover tools that are used in healthcare quality.

1. Brainstorm:

Brainstorming is a widely recognized technique for generating creative ideas and solutions. It involves the free-flow generation of ideas without immediate evaluation or judgment, which can foster excitement and encourage the involvement of all group members (Osborn, 1963). This method allows participants to build upon each other's ideas, leading to innovative solutions to problems (Paulus & Kenworthy, 2019).

One of the key aspects of brainstorming is that it encourages the free involvement of all members. By suspending judgment during the idea generation phase, participants feel more comfortable sharing their thoughts, which can lead to a more diverse range of ideas (Gogus, 2012). This non-evaluative environment is crucial for maximizing creativity and ensuring that all voices are heard.

Brainstorming sessions are typically used when a list of possible ideas is needed. This approach can be particularly effective in situations where original solutions are required, as it allows for the combination and improvement of ideas (Baruah & Paulus, 2008). The process of building upon each other's ideas can result in more refined and effective solutions than those generated by individuals working alone (Brown & Paulus, 2002).

In summary, brainstorming is a valuable tool for generating a wide range of ideas and fostering creativity within a group. By encouraging free-flowing idea generation and suspending judgment, it can lead to innovative solutions and greater involvement from all participants.

2. Multi-voting:

Multi-voting is a structured decision-making process used to determine the most popular or important items from a list, often without extensive discussion. This method is particularly useful in group settings where consensus is needed, and it helps to narrow down a large list of options to a manageable number (Linderman, 2006).

In a multi-voting session, each member of the group identifies the items they consider most important from the original list. These selections are then scored, and items with the lowest scores are eliminated. This process is repeated until the item or solution with the highest priority is identified (Tague, 2005). The simplicity and efficiency of multi-voting make it an effective tool for prioritizing options and reaching group consensus (Brassard & Ritter, 1994).

Multi-voting is particularly beneficial in situations where a large number of ideas or options need to be evaluated quickly. By focusing on the most important items and eliminating less critical ones, the group can efficiently identify the top priorities (Linderman, 2006). This method also ensures that all members have a voice in the decision-making process, which can enhance group cohesion and commitment to the final decision (Tague, 2005).

Multi-voting can be illustrated with the example of selecting an employee of the month. Suppose the candidates are Wafa, Taleen, Yara, Abdulrahman, and Mohammed. Each member of the group votes for the candidates they believe should be nominated. The votes are as follows:

In this scenario, **Abdulrahman** receives the highest number of votes (5), making him the top candidate for employee of the month. **Wafa** and **Mohammed**, with 4 votes each, are also strong contenders. Taleen and Yara get (3) votes. This process helps the group quickly identify the most popular choices without extensive discussion, ensuring an efficient and democratic decision-making process.

Table 8.1: Multi-voting of the employee of the month

Employee	Votes	Total
Wafa	✓✓✓✓	4 🥈
Abdulrahman	✓✓✓✓✓	5 🏆 🥇
Taleen	✓✓✓	3 🥉
Yara	✓✓✓	3 🥉
Mohammed	✓✓✓✓	4 🥈

3. Delphi methodology:

The Delphi Method is a structured communication technique originally developed as a systematic, interactive forecasting method which relies on a panel of experts. It is particularly useful for situations where the members of a group are not in the same location, making it a virtual method of consensus-building. This method combines brainstorming and multi-voting techniques to gather and refine expert opinions through multiple rounds of questionnaires, often conducted via mail or email when in-person meetings are not feasible (Khodyakov et al., 2023).

The process begins with the selection of a panel of experts who are asked to respond to a series of questionnaires. After each round, a facilitator provides an anonymized summary of the experts' forecasts and reasons. The experts are encouraged to revise their earlier answers in light of the replies of other members of their panel. This process is repeated until the group reaches a consensus or the responses stabilize (Niederberger & Renn, 2023).

The Delphi Method has been widely used in various fields, including health sciences, social sciences, and technology. It is particularly valued for its ability to harness the collective intelligence of a group while minimizing the influence of dominant individuals and reducing the effects of groupthink (Khodyakov et al., 2023). This method is also adaptable to virtual environments, making it a practical tool for remote collaboration and decision-making.

4. Flow chart:

A flow chart is a visual representation that outlines the steps of a process in a sequential manner. It is particularly useful for identifying the ideal paths that a product or service follows, which helps in pinpointing any deviations from the expected process. Flow charts are widely used for documenting programs and processes, providing a clear and concise way to examine how various steps are interconnected (Vu-Ngoc et al., 2018).

Flow charts typically use standardized symbols to represent different types of actions or steps in a process. For example, rectangles are used to denote process steps, diamonds indicate decision points, and arrows show the flow of the process. This visual format makes it easier to understand complex processes at a glance and can be an invaluable tool for both analysis and communication (Vu-Ngoc et al., 2018).

Common Flow Chart Symbols

- **Oval**: Represents the start or end of a process.
- **Rectangle**: Indicates a process step or action.
- **Diamond**: Denotes a decision point, where the process can branch based on a yes/no question or condition.
- **Arrow**: Shows the direction of the flow from one step to the next.

Figure 8.1: Flow chart

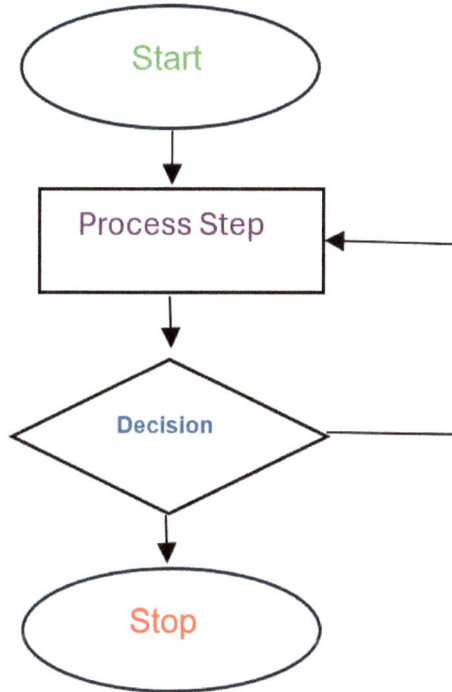

These symbols help in creating a clear and standardized visual representation of a process, making it easier to understand and communicate complex workflows (Bianconi, 2024).

1. Process Map:

Process mapping in healthcare involves creating a visual representation of the steps involved in a healthcare process. This helps to identify inefficiencies, redundancies, and opportunities for improvement. According to Antonacci et al. (2021), process mapping supports better understanding of complex systems and adaptation of improvement interventions to their local context. The study outlines a conceptual framework for process mapping in healthcare, which includes preparation, planning, data gathering, map generation, analysis, and implementation (Antonacci et al., 2021).

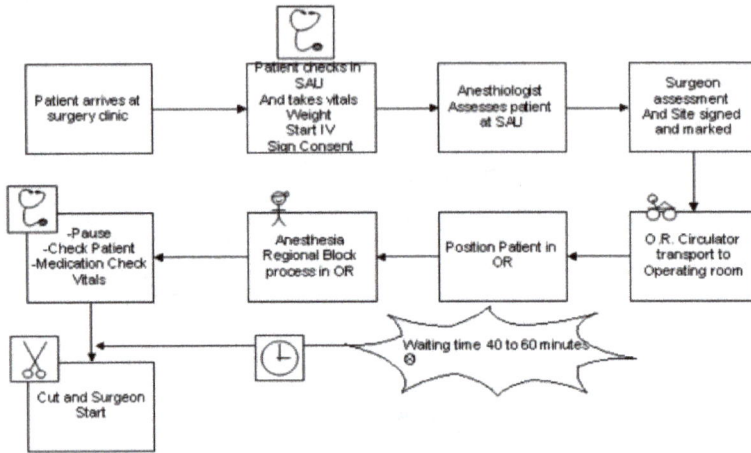

Figure 8.2: Process Map (Abduljawad, 2021)

2. Check Sheets:

Check sheets are a fundamental quality tool used to gather data based on sample observations, which helps in detecting patterns and trends. This tool is particularly useful at the beginning of most problem-solving cycles, as it provides a logical starting point for data collection and analysis.

In healthcare, check sheets are designed to systematically record data, making it easier to identify trends, frequencies, and distributions. They are commonly used in various quality control and process improvement activities. For instance, check sheets can record the frequency of medication errors in a hospital setting, helping to pinpoint areas that need improvement (Basu, 2023).

3. Pareto Chart:

A Pareto chart is a specialized bar graph that displays a series of bars arranged in descending order of their height from left to right. This visual representation helps to identify the most significant factors in a dataset by showing the frequency or impact of causes. The height of each bar reflects the frequency of occurrence or the impact of the cause, emphasizing the importance of each factor.

The Pareto principle, also known as the 80/20 rule, underpins the use of Pareto charts. This principle suggests that approximately 80% of the effects come from 20% of the possible causes. By focusing on these "vital few" causes, organizations can achieve significant improvements more efficiently (Alkiayat, 2021).

Example of a Pareto Chart in Healthcare: 2 vital few departments out of 10 (Emergency and ICU) had 80% of deaths.

Table 8.2: Five Year Crude Mortality rates by clinical department at hospital X

Hospital Department	# of deaths	Cumulative Total	Cumulative %
ED	520	520	42%
ICU	473	993	80%
Oncology	72	1065	85%
Neuro surgery	61	1126	90%
Cardiac Surgery	53	1179	94%
General surgery	24	1203	96%
Pediatrics	18	1221	98%
Orthopedic Surgery	11	1232	99%
Gastroenterology	9	1241	99%
Nephrology	8	1249	100%
Ophthalmology	0	1249	100%
Dental	0	1249	100%
Total	1249		

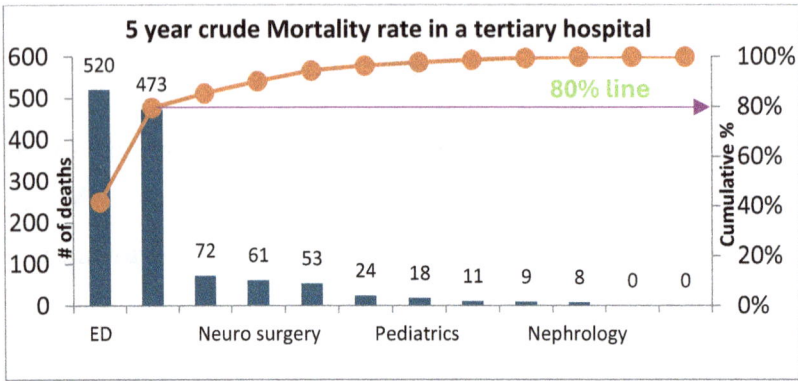

Figure 8.3 : Pareto Chart 5 year Crude Mortality rates by department at hospital X

4. Bar graph and histogram:

Bar Graph:

A bar graph is used to compare different categories of data. It displays discrete data using rectangular bars, where each bar represents a category, and the length of the bar corresponds to the value or frequency of that category. The bars in a bar graph are separated by spaces to emphasize that the categories are distinct and not continuous (Basu, 2023).

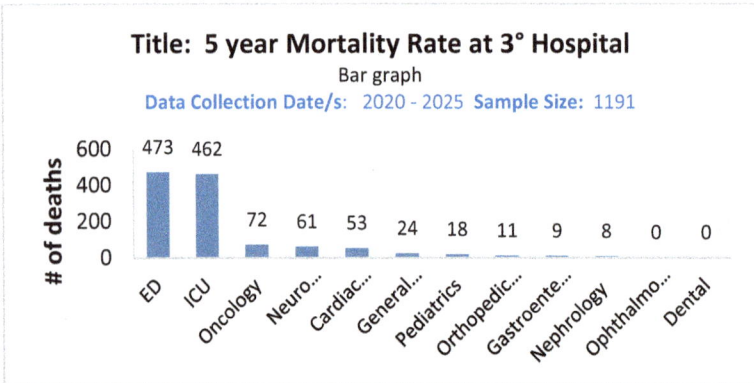

Figure 8.4: Bar graph of the number of deaths by department

Histogram:

A histogram, on the other hand, is used to represent the frequency distribution of continuous data. It displays data in adjacent bars, where each bar represents a range of values (or bins of **grouped data**), and the height of the bar corresponds to the frequency of data points within that range. Unlike bar graphs, the bars in a histogram touch each other to indicate that the data is continuous (Basu, 2023).

Table 8.3 Number of patients of each age group at hospital Z

Age group	No. of patients
0 - 10	15
11 - 20	25
21 - 30	40
31 - 40	30
41 - 50	20
51 - 60	10
61 - 70	5
71 - 80	3

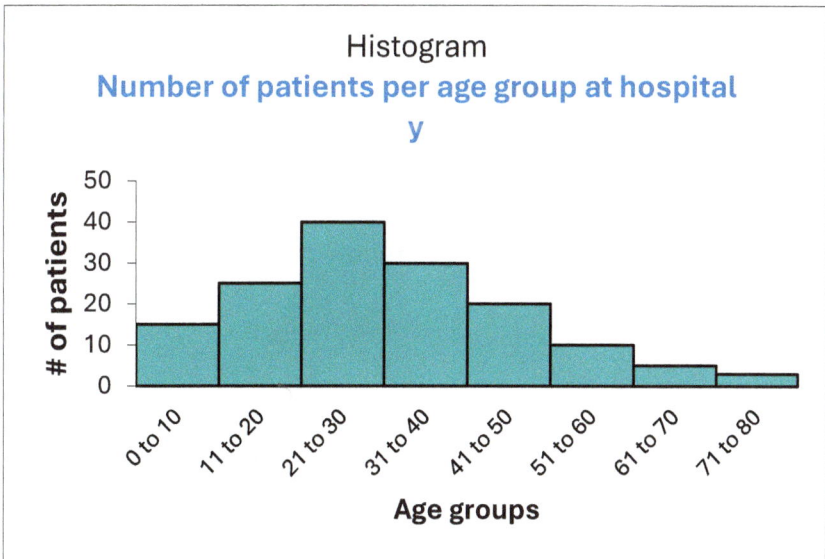

Figure 8.5 : An example of a histogram

Key Differences:

1. **Data Type:**

   o   **Bar Graph**: Compares discrete categories of data.

o **Histogram**: Represents the frequency distribution of continuous data.

2. **Bar Spacing:**

   o **Bar Graph**: Bars are separated by spaces.
   o **Histogram**: Bars are adjacent with no spaces between them.

3. **Purpose:**

   o **Bar Graph**: Used to compare different categories.
   o **Histogram**: Used to show the distribution of a dataset.

4. **Reordering:**

   o **Bar Graph**: Bars can be reordered.
   o **Histogram**: Bars are ordered by the range of values.

Example

- **Bar Graph**: Comparing the number of patient deaths in different departments of a hospital.
- **Histogram**: Showing the distribution of patient wait times in the emergency department.

5. Pie Chart:

A pie chart is a circular statistical graphic divided into slices to illustrate numerical proportions. Each slice of the pie represents a category's contribution to the whole, with the arc length of each slice proportional to the quantity it represents (Basu, 2023).

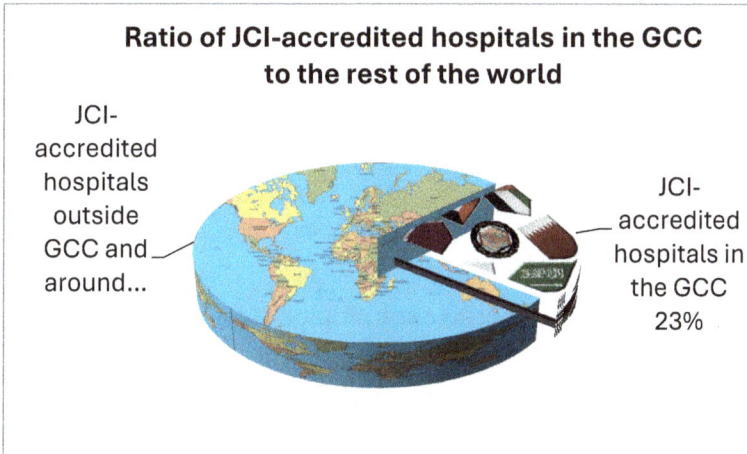

Figure 8.6: Pie chart (Abduljawad, 2013)

6. Cause and effect diagram or Ishakawa fishbone:

A cause and effect diagram, also known as an Ishikawa or fishbone diagram, is a tool used to systematically identify and analyze the root causes of a specific problem or effect. This diagram helps in organizing potential causes into categories, making it easier to understand the complex interplay of factors contributing to an issue (Coccia, 2018).

The structure of a Fishbone Diagram resembles the skeleton of a fish, with the main problem or effect at the "head" and the causes extending as "bones" along the spine. Each major cause is represented as a branch off the spine, with sub-causes branching off from these main causes. This hierarchical structure helps in breaking down the problem into manageable parts (Wong, 2011).

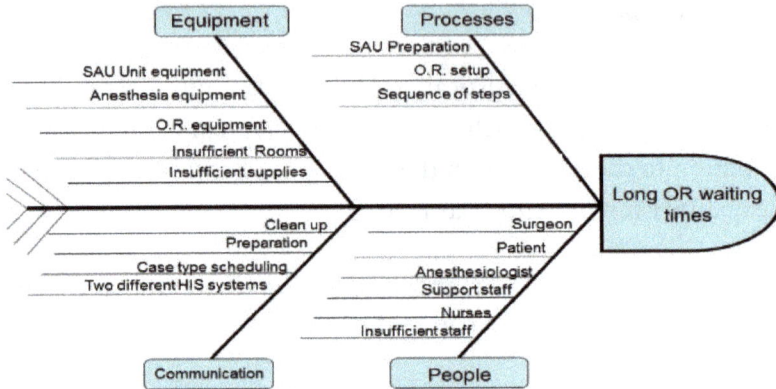

Figure 8.7: Ishikawa fish bone (Cause and effect diagram) of long turnover times (Abduljawad, 2021).

7. Scatter diagrams:

A scatter diagram, also known as a scatter plot, is a graphical representation used to display the relationship between two numerical variables. Each point on the scatter diagram represents the values of two variables, with the x-coordinate representing the independent variable and the y-coordinate representing the dependent variable.

An example would be Studying the Relationship Between Study Hours and Test Scores

- **Independent Variable**: Hours of study. This is the variable that you can control or change to see how it affects the outcome.
- **Dependent Variable**: Test scores. This is the variable that you measure to see if it changes based on the hours of study.

Another clinical example the effect of a new medication on blood pressure

- **Independent Variable:** The new medication being administered. This is the variable that the researcher manipulates to observe its effect.
- **Dependent Variable:** The patients' blood pressure levels. This is the variable that is measured to see if it changes in response to the independent variable. (Basu, 2023).

Types of Scatter Diagrams

1. **Positive Correlation**:
   - **Description**: As one variable increases, the other variable also increases.
   - **Example**: Total number of hours studied for the SMLE and the final score.

Table 8.4 Number of hours studied and corresponding SMLE Score.

No. of hours studied	SMLE score
0	0
1	10
2	15
3	20
4	25
5	30
6	35
7	40
8	45
9	50
10	55
11	60
12	65
13	70
14	75
15	80
16	85
17	90
18	95
19	97
20	100

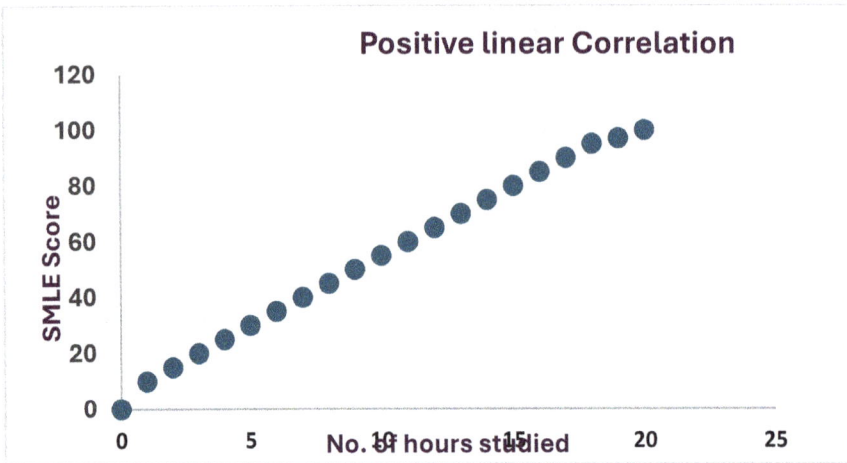

Figure 8.8 Positive Correlation Scatter plot

o **Visualization**: Points form an upward-sloping pattern from left to right.

2. **Negative Correlation:**
   o **Description**: As one variable increases, the other variable decreases.
   o **Example**: The number of hours spent watching TV and grades in school. More TV time is often associated with lower grades.

Table 8.5 Number of hours watched TV and SDLE Score

No. of hours studied	SDLE score
0	100
1	97
2	95
3	90
4	85
5	80
6	75
7	70
8	65
9	60
10	55
11	50
12	45
13	40
14	35
15	30
16	25
17	20
18	15
19	10
20	0

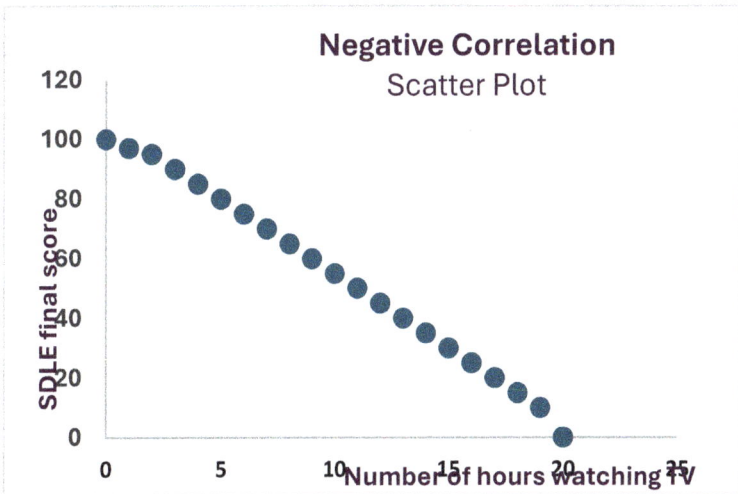

Figure 8.9 Negative correlation scatter plot

- o **Visualization**: Points form a downward-sloping pattern from left to right.

2. **No Correlation**:
   - o **Description**: There is no apparent relationship between the variables.
   - o **Example**: Foot size and test score. There is no direct relationship between these two variables.

Table 8.6 Foot size in inches and Aptitude test score

Foot Size	Test score
5.91	22.32
5.29	69.64
9.71	2.7
8.67	82.69
11.4	41.91
9.08	45.97
8.86	12.45
5.27	58.68
6.56	89.55
9.91	68.34
10.23	4.25
10.78	94.39
5.83	89.96
10.94	45.97
6.21	89.21
8.59	43.43
7.42	15.07
9.67	51.66
11.71	86.77
7.92	37.97

Figure 8.10 No correlation scatter plot

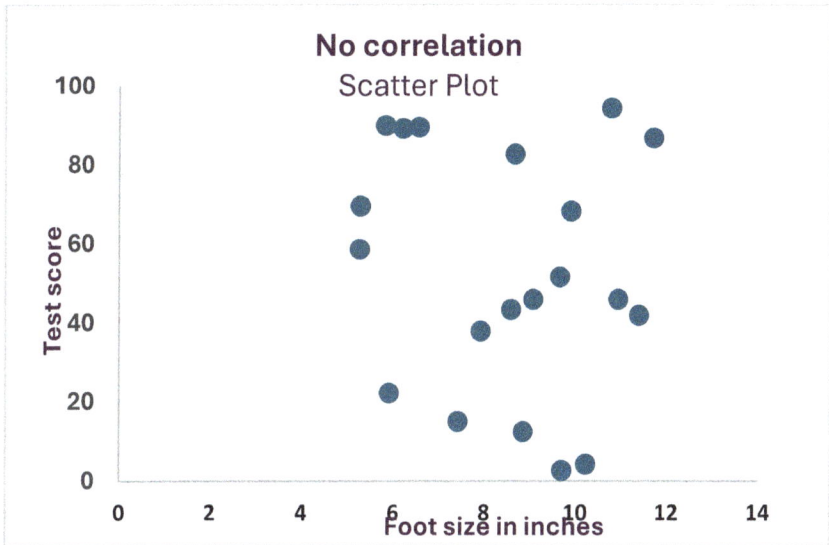

o   **Visualization**: Points are scattered randomly without any discernible pattern.

1) Run Chart:

A run chart is a fundamental tool in quality improvement that graphically displays data points over time. This visual representation helps in identifying trends, shifts, or patterns in the data, which are crucial for process improvement activities (Perla et al., 2011). The y-axis of a run chart is labeled with the variable being measured, while the x-axis is labeled with time intervals (Winckler et al., 2024).

A key feature of a run chart is the mean line, which represents the average value of the plotted data points. This line helps in distinguishing between common cause variation (natural variation inherent in the process) and special cause variation (variation due to specific changes or interventions) (Perla et al., 2011). By analyzing the data points in relation to the mean line, one can observe trends, such as six or seven consecutive points moving in the same direction, which indicates a non-random pattern (Winckler et al., 2024).Run charts are particularly useful for displaying variation in data and for monitoring the impact of process improvement activities. For instance, they can show whether changes implemented in a process lead to sustained improvements over time (Perla et al., 2011). This makes run charts an essential tool for continuous quality improvement in various fields, including healthcare, manufacturing, and service industries (Winckler et al., 2024).

Table 8.7 Number of hospital patient falls from Jan-Dec 2024

Date of Observation	# of patient falls
Jan-24	5
Feb-24	7
Mar-24	6
Apr-24	4
May-24	8
Jun-24	5
Jul-24	3
Aug-24	6
Sep-24	4
Oct-24	7
Nov-24	5
Dec-24	3

Figure 8.11 Run Chart of hospital patient falls during 2024

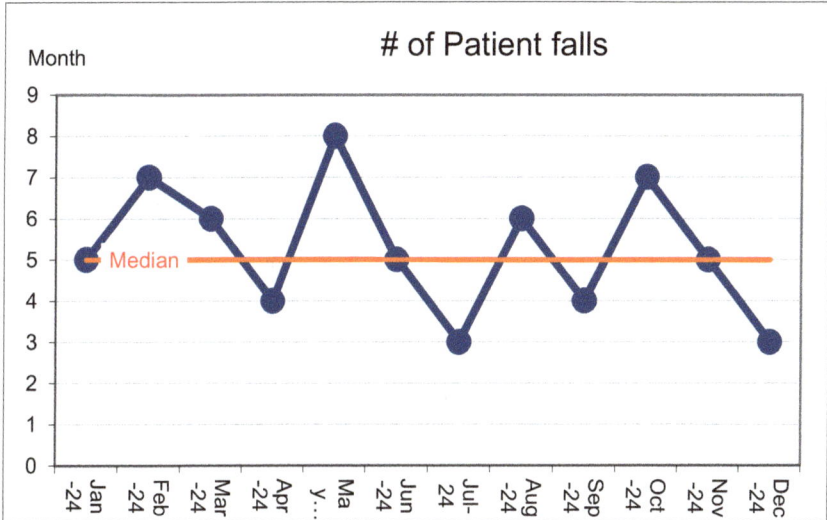

2) Control Charts:

Control charts are essential tools in statistical process control, used to monitor the stability of processes over time. They include control limits, specifically the Upper Control Limit (UCL) and Lower Control Limit (LCL), which are set above and below the mean line. These limits are typically calculated by adding and subtracting three standard deviations from the mean of the data (Montgomery, 2020).

Common Cause Variation

Common cause variation is inherent to the process and is random. It is observed on control charts as points that fall between the control limits without any specific pattern (Benneyan et al., 2003). This type of variation is due to the natural fluctuations in the process and should not be immediately fixed. Instead, management should focus on identifying and understanding the root causes before attempting to eliminate them (Montgomery, 2020). The recordings will be between the UCL and LCL.

Figure 8.12 Common cause variation (Monthly Inpatient falls between Jan 2023- Jan 2025)

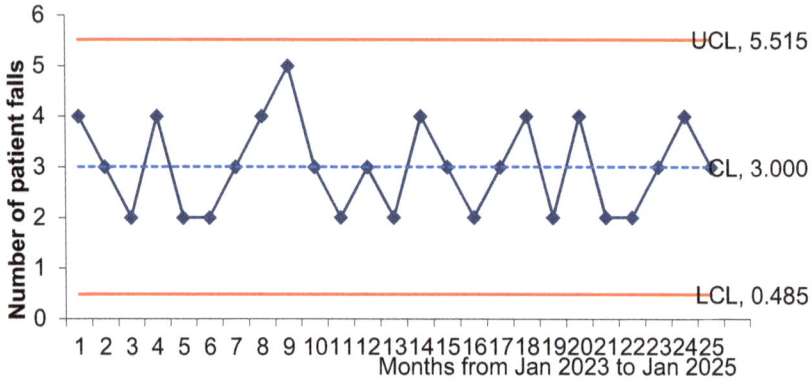

Special Cause Variation

Special cause variation, on the other hand, is not inherent to the process. It is observed as any point outside the control limits or within the limits but exhibiting special patterns (Thor et al., 2004). This type of variation indicates that something unusual has occurred in the process, and it should be addressed by employees as soon as it is observed (Benneyan et al., 2003). Some readings will be outside the UCL or LCL.

Figure 8.13 Special cause variation (Monthly Inpatient falls between Jan

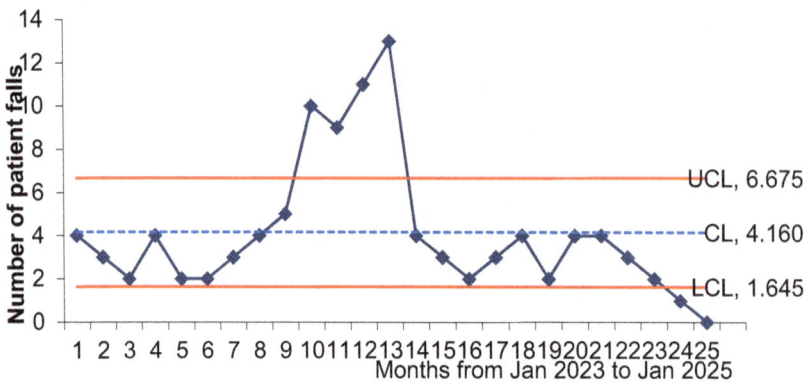

2023- Jan 2025)

Common versus Special cause variation simplified:

Common cause versus special cause variation can be illustrated by the daily commute from Jeddah to Makkah. If the average commute time ranges between 50 and 60 minutes, variations within 5 minutes (i.e., $10 \div 4 = 2.5$ minutes is 1 standard deviation (SD); 2 SDs = 5 minutes) are considered common cause variations. These variations might result from factors such as stopping at a red light for a bit longer than anticipated, driving slightly faster or slower than usual, or stopping at a checkpoint. However, if the commute time exceeds 2 standard deviations (i.e., more than 66 minutes or less than 44 minutes), this is considered special cause variation. Special causes could include adverse weather conditions, such as rain, schools being on vacation, or a significant accident causing extreme traffic delays.

Special Patterns in a Control Chart

Special patterns in a control chart include a run of seven or more points above or below the mean line, a run of 14 points in a zigzag pattern above and below the central line, two consecutive points near the UCL or LCL, and any point outside the UCL or LCL (Thor et al., 2004). These patterns indicate non-random variation and suggest that the process may be out of control, requiring immediate investigation and corrective action (Montgomery, 2020).

References:

1. ABDULJAWAD, A. A. (2021). Reducing turnover time in the orthopedic department operating room at a tertiary hospital. Journal of Complementary Medicine Research, 12(4), 126-126.
2. Abduljawad, A. (2013). Impact of accreditation on the quality of hospitals in the Gulf Cooperation Council countries. The University of Oklahoma Health Sciences Center.
3. Alkiayat, M. (2021). A practical guide to creating a Pareto chart as a quality improvement tool. Global Journal on Quality and Safety in Healthcare, 4(2), 83-84. https://doi.org/10.36401/JQSH-21-X1
4. Antonacci, G., Lennox, L., Barlow, J., Evans, L., & Reed, J. (2021). Process mapping in healthcare: A systematic review. *BMC Health Services Research, 21*(1), 342. https://doi.org/10.1186/s12913-021-06254-1
5. Baruah, J., & Paulus, P. B. (2008). Effects of training on idea generation in groups. Small Group Research, 39(5), 523-541.
6. Basu, R. (2023). Quality Management: Tools and Techniques. Springer. https://doi.org/10.1007/978-3-030-56789-1
7. Benneyan, J. C., Lloyd, R. C., & Plsek, P. E. (2003). Statistical process control as a tool for research and healthcare improvement. Quality and Safety in Health Care, 12(6), 458-464. https://doi.org/10.1136/qhc.12.6.458
8. Bianconi, F. (2024). Flowcharts. In Data and Process Visualisation for Graphic Communication. Springer. https://doi.org/10.1007/978-3-031-57051-3_12
9. Brown, V. R., & Paulus, P. B. (2002). Making group brainstorming more effective: Recommendations from an associative memory perspective. Current Directions in Psychological Science, 11(6), 208-212.
10. Coccia, M. (2018). The Fishbone Diagram to Identify, Systematize and Analyze the Sources of General Purpose Technologies. Journal of Social and Administrative Sciences, 4(4), 291-303. https://doi.org/10.2139/ssrn.3100011
11. Gogus, A. (2012). Brainstorming and learning. In N. M. Seel (Ed.), Encyclopedia of the Sciences of Learning (pp. 484-488). Springer.
12. Khodyakov, D., Grant, S., Kroger, J., Gadwah-Meaden, C., Motala, A., & Larkin, J. (2023). Disciplinary trends in the use of the Delphi method: A bibliometric analysis. PLOS ONE, 18(8), e0289009. https://doi.org/10.1371/journal.pone.0289009

13. Montgomery, D. C. (2020). Introduction to Statistical Quality Control (8th ed.). Wiley.

14. Niederberger, M., & Renn, O. (2023). Delphi Methods In The Social And Health Sciences: Concepts, applications and case studies. Springer. https://doi.org/10.1007/978-3-658-38862-1

15. Osborn, A. F. (1963). Applied imagination: Principles and procedures of creative problem-solving (3rd ed.). Scribner.

16. Paulus, P. B., & Kenworthy, J. B. (2019). Effective brainstorming. In P. B. Paulus & B. A. Nijstad (Eds.), The Oxford handbook of group creativity and innovation (pp. 286-305). Oxford University Press.

17. Perla, R. J., Provost, L. P., & Murray, S. K. (2011). The run chart: A simple analytical tool for learning from variation in healthcare processes. BMJ Quality & Safety, 20(1), 46-51. https://doi.org/10.1136/bmjqs.2009.037895

18. Thor, J., Lundberg, J., Ask, J., Olsson, J., Carli, C., Harenstam, K. P., & Brommels, M. (2004). Application of statistical process control in healthcare improvement: Systematic review. Quality and Safety in Health Care, 13(4), 247-253. https://doi.org/10.1136/qshc.2003.007641

19. Vu-Ngoc, H., Elawady, S. S., Mehyar, G. M., Abdelhamid, A. H., Mattar, O. M., & Halhouli, O. (2018). Quality of flow diagram in systematic review and/or meta-analysis. PLOS ONE, 13(6), e0195955. https://doi.org/10.1371/journal.pone.0195955

20. Winckler, B., McKenzie, S., & Lo, H. (2024). A practical guide to QI data analysis: Run and statistical process control charts. Hospital Pediatrics, 14(1), e83-e89. https://doi.org/10.1542/hpeds.2023-007296

21. Wong, K. C. (2011). Using an Ishikawa diagram as a tool to assist memory and retrieval of relevant medical cases from the medical literature. Journal of Medical Case Reports, 5, 120. https://doi.org/10.1186/1752-1947-5-120

Chapter 9

Statistics in Healthcare Quality

Data, information, and knowledge:

Data, information, and knowledge are interconnected concepts that play crucial roles in various fields, including information science, data science, and knowledge management. Understanding the distinctions and relationships among these concepts is essential for effectively managing and utilizing data.

Data refers to raw, unprocessed facts and figures without context. These can be numbers, characters, images, or other outputs from devices that collect information. Data on its own has no meaning until it is processed and interpreted (Rowley, 2007).

Information is data that has been processed, organized, or structured in a way that adds meaning. Information is essentially data that has been given context and relevance, making it useful for decision-making. For example, a dataset containing temperatures recorded over a month becomes information when it is organized to show trends or patterns (Ackoff, 1989).

Knowledge is derived from information by applying rules, context, and experience. It involves the synthesis of information to form judgments, insights, and predictions. Knowledge is often categorized into explicit knowledge, which can be easily communicated and documented, and tacit knowledge, which is personal and harder to formalize (Nonaka & Takeuchi, 1995).

The transformation from data to information to knowledge involves several processes, including data collection, data processing, information dissemination, and knowledge application. This transformation is critical in fields such as business intelligence, where raw data is analyzed to produce actionable insights (Davenport & Prusak, 1998).

Types of Data:

Continuous Data

Continuous data can be divided into two main types: interval and ratio data. Both types are essential in various fields, including healthcare, social sciences, and natural sciences, due to their ability to represent and analyze quantitative measurements.

Interval Data

Interval data is a type of continuous data where the difference between any two values is meaningful and equal. This type of data does not have a true zero point, meaning that zero does not indicate the absence of the quantity being measured. Common examples of interval data include temperature scales like Celsius and Fahrenheit, where the difference between degrees is consistent, but zero does not mean the absence of temperature (Stevens, 1946). For instance, the difference between 10°C and 20°C is the same as the difference between 20°C and 30°C. However, 0°C does not imply 'no temperature'; it is simply another point on the scale. This characteristic makes interval data useful for measuring variables where relative differences are important, but absolute comparisons are not (Velleman & Wilkinson, 1993).

Other examples of interval data include IQ scores and standardized test scores. IQ scores, for instance, have consistent intervals between values, but an IQ of zero does not mean the absence of intelligence. Similarly, standardized test scores, such as SAT scores, have equal intervals between scores, but a score of zero does not indicate a complete lack of knowledge or ability (Lewis-Beck, Bryman, & Liao, 2004).

Ratio Data

Ratio data is another type of continuous data, but unlike interval data, it has a true zero point, which indicates the absence of the quantity being measured. This allows for meaningful comparisons using multiplication and division. Examples of ratio data include weight, height, and time, where zero represents none of the quantity (Stevens, 1946). In healthcare, the nurse-to-patient ratio in an ICU is a practical example of ratio data. If there is a 1:2 nurse-to-patient ratio, it means one nurse is responsible for two patients. This ratio can be scaled up or down, and zero would mean no nurses or no patients, making the zero point meaningful (Polit & Beck, 2017).

Other examples of ratio data include age and income. Age is measured from a defined point of starting, which is birth (age 0). If someone is 20 years old, they are twice as old as someone who is 10 years old. Income, on the other hand, can be measured in currency units, where zero income means no earnings, and an income of 100,000 Saudi Riyals is twice as much as 50,000 Riyals (Katz, 2006).

Categorical Data:

Categorical data can be divided into two main types: nominal and ordinal data. Both types are essential in various fields, including healthcare, social sciences, and market research, due to their ability to categorize and analyze qualitative information.

Nominal Data

Nominal data is a type of categorical data that represents variables with no inherent order or ranking among the categories. This type of data is used to label variables without providing any quantitative value. Nominal data is often used in various fields to categorize and analyze qualitative information.

Examples of Nominal Data

1. **Surgical Patients**: In a hospital setting, patients can be categorized based on their surgical status. For example:

- o 1: Pre-operative (Pre-op)
- o 2: Post-operative (Post-op) These categories are used to differentiate between patients who are awaiting surgery and those who have already undergone surgery. There is no inherent order between these categories; they are simply labels used for classification (Polit & Beck, 2017).

2. **Gender**: Gender is another common example of nominal data. Traditionally, gender has been categorized as:

- o 1: Male (M)
- o 2: Female (F) These categories are used to identify the gender of individuals without implying any order or ranking. In modern contexts, additional categories such as non-binary or other may also be included (Lewis-Beck, Bryman, & Liao, 2004).

3. **Blood Type**: Blood types are categorized nominally as:

- o A
- o B
- o AB
- o O These categories are used to identify different blood groups without any inherent ranking among them (Katz, 2006).

4. **Marital Status**: Marital status can be categorized as:

- o Single
- o Married
- o Divorced
- o Widowed These categories are used to describe the marital status of individuals without any implied order (Babbie, Halley, & Zaino, 2007).

Ordinal Data

Ordinal data is another type of categorical data, but unlike nominal data, it has a meaningful order or ranking among the categories. This type of data is used to represent variables where the order matters, but the differences between the categories are not necessarily equal.

Examples of Ordinal Data

1. **Education Level**: Education level is a common example of ordinal data. The categories are:

   o Diploma
   o Bachelor's Degree (BSc)
   o Master's Degree (MS)
   o Doctorate (PhD) These categories are ordered in a meaningful way, indicating increasing levels of education. However, the differences between these levels are not necessarily equal (Stevens, 1946).

2. **Socioeconomic Status**: Socioeconomic status can be categorized as:

   o Low
   o Middle
   o High These categories indicate an order from low to high socioeconomic status, but the intervals between these categories are not equal (Velleman & Wilkinson, 1993).

3. **Pain Severity**: Pain severity is often measured on an ordinal scale with categories such as:

   o Mild
   o Moderate
   o Severe These categories indicate increasing levels of pain, but the differences between these levels are not equal (Babbie et al., 2007).

4. **Job Satisfaction**: Job satisfaction can be categorized as:

   o Very Dissatisfied
   o Dissatisfied
   o Neutral
   o Satisfied
   o Very Satisfied These categories are ordered to reflect increasing levels of satisfaction, but the intervals between these categories are not equal (Lewis-Beck et al., 2004).

Comparing the Power of Categorical and Continuous Data

When comparing the power of categorical (qualitative) data and continuous (quantitative) data, continuous data is generally considered more powerful statistically. This difference in power stems from the nature of the data and the types of analyses that can be performed.

Categorical Data (Qualitative)

Categorical data, also known as qualitative data, includes variables that can be divided into distinct groups or categories. Examples include gender, blood type, and marital status. The primary limitation of categorical data is that it does not provide information about the magnitude or order of differences between categories. This restricts the types of statistical analyses that can be performed, often limiting them to non-parametric methods such as chi-square tests or frequency counts (Stevens, 1946).

Because categorical data lacks numerical value and order, it is less powerful in detecting subtle differences and relationships within the data. For instance, while you can count the number of males and females in a sample, you cannot measure the degree of difference between these categories (Polit & Beck, 2017).

Continuous Data (Quantitative)

Continuous data, or quantitative data, represents variables that can take on an infinite number of values within a given range. Examples include weight, height, temperature, and income. Continuous data is more powerful statistically because it allows for a wide range of mathematical operations and statistical analyses, including measures of central tendency (mean, median, mode), variability (standard deviation, variance), and more complex analyses like regression and correlation (Velleman & Wilkinson, 1993).

The key advantage of continuous data is its ability to provide detailed and precise measurements. This allows for the detection of subtle differences and relationships within the data. For example, continuous data can show not only that one person is taller than another but also by how much, and it can quantify the relationship between height and weight (Katz, 2006).

Sampling

Sampling is a fundamental concept in research methodology, involving the selection of a subset of individuals from a larger population to represent that population. This process allows researchers to make inferences about the entire population without needing to study every individual.

Population

A population is the total aggregate or group of cases that meet a designated set of criteria for inclusion in a study. It encompasses all individuals or items that possess the characteristics of interest to the researcher (Polit & Beck, 2017). Examples of populations in healthcare research might include:

- All physicians
- All nurses
- All patients who have expired at Hospital A
- Nurses or risk managers under the age of 40 years

Sample

A sample is a subset of the population selected for the actual study. The purpose of sampling is to draw conclusions about the population based on the data collected from the sample. Sampling is essential because it is often impractical or impossible to collect data from every member of a population (Creswell & Creswell, 2018).

How Do Researchers Sample?

Sampling is a critical process in research methodology, allowing researchers to draw conclusions about a population based on a subset of that population. There are various types of sampling methods, each with its own strengths and applications.

Types of Sampling

Probability Sampling

Probability sampling requires that every element in the population has an equal or random chance of being selected in the sample. This method is essential for ensuring that the sample is representative of the population, thereby allowing for generalizable and unbiased results (Creswell & Creswell, 2018).

Simple Random Sampling

Simple random sampling is a type of probability sampling where all subjects in the population have an equal chance of being chosen. This method is straightforward and ensures that every individual has the same probability of selection.

Example: Pulling out a name from a hat that contains all possible names is a classic example of simple random sampling. This method ensures that each name has an equal chance of being selected (Polit & Beck, 2017).

Systematic Sampling

Systematic sampling involves drawing or selecting every nth element from the population. This method is useful when a complete list of the population is available and can be systematically ordered.

Example: Picking every third name from a list of possible names is an example of systematic sampling. This method ensures a systematic approach to selection, which can be easier to implement than simple random sampling (Katz, 2006).

Stratified Random Sampling

Stratified random sampling involves dividing the population into homogeneous groups or subpopulations (strata) and then randomly selecting samples from each stratum. This method ensures that specific subgroups are adequately represented within the sample.

Example: Dividing the population into 13 regions of the Kingdom of Saudi Arabia (KSA) or the 7 emirates of the United Arab Emirates (UAE) and then randomly selecting individuals from each region or emirate ensures that each subgroup is represented (Polit & Beck, 2017).

Cluster Sampling

Cluster sampling involves dividing the population into clusters or groups and then randomly selecting entire clusters for study. This method is useful when the population is too large and dispersed for simple random sampling.

Example: Dividing the population into 13 regions of the KSA and then clustering the samples into medical schools in the Mekkah region. Further clustering could involve selecting specific cities such as Mekkah, Jeddah, Taif, Leeth, Albaha, and Qunfutha (Creswell & Creswell, 2018).

Non-Probability Sampling

Non-probability sampling is a sampling technique where there is no way of estimating the probability that each element will be included in the sample. This method is often used when it is impractical or impossible to conduct probability sampling. However, it comes with significant drawbacks, particularly in terms of the generalizability of the results.

Drawbacks of Non-Probability Sampling

The primary drawback of non-probability sampling is that the results cannot be generalized to the population. This limitation arises because the sample may not be representative of the population, leading to selection bias. For example, if a researcher uses convenience sampling to survey students in a single university, the findings may not be applicable to students in other universities (Etikan, Musa, & Alkassim, 2016).

Types of Non-Probability Sampling

Convenience Sampling

Convenience sampling involves selecting any available group of subjects. This approach is often used for its ease and speed, but it is prone to significant bias because the sample may not be representative of the population.

Example: Surveying people at a shopping mall to understand consumer behavior. The sample is convenient but may not represent the broader population (Bornstein, Jager, & Putnick, 2013).

Snowball Sampling

Snowball sampling is a type of convenience sampling where existing study subjects recruit future subjects from among their acquaintances. This method is useful for studying populations that are difficult to identify, but it can introduce selection bias.

Example: Sending a survey to a list of members of an organization that represents doctors, who then forward the survey to other doctors they know. Similarly, sending a survey to a list of members of a nursing organization (Naderifar, Goli, & Ghaljaie, 2017).

Expert Sampling

Expert sampling involves selecting individuals with specific expertise in the area of study. This method is often used in the Delphi technique, where experts provide insights based on their knowledge.

Example: Selecting a panel of climate scientists to provide predictions about future climate trends. The sample is based on expertise rather than random selection (Baker, Brick, Bates, Battaglia, Couper et al., 2013).

Quota Sampling

Quota sampling involves pre-specifying characteristics of the sample and determining the proportions of elements needed from various segments of the population. This method ensures that specific subgroups are represented in the sample.

Example: Sampling 5% or 30 cases, whichever is greater, from each department in a company to ensure representation from all departments (Daniel, 2012).

Disadvantages of Non-Probability Sampling

The main disadvantage of non-probability sampling is the inability to generalize the results to the entire population. This limitation is due to the potential for selection bias, as the sample may not accurately reflect the diversity of the population. For instance, in snowball sampling, those who agree to participate may differ significantly from those who do not, leading to biased results (Etikan et al., 2016).

Sample Size Factors

Determining the appropriate sample size for a study is crucial for ensuring the validity and reliability of the research findings. Several factors influence the determination of sample size, including the research purpose, the design, the level of confidence desired, the anticipated degree of difference between study groups, and the size of the population (Creswell & Creswell, 2018).

Factors Influencing Sample Size

- **Research Purpose**: The objectives of the study significantly impact the sample size. Exploratory studies may require smaller samples, while confirmatory studies aimed at testing specific hypotheses often need larger samples to achieve sufficient statistical power (Faber & Fonseca, 2014).
- **Research Design**: The complexity of the research design also affects sample size. Studies with multiple groups or variables typically require larger samples to ensure adequate power for detecting differences or relationships (Kadam & Bhalerao, 2010).
- **Level of Confidence**: The desired level of confidence, often set at 95% or 99%, determines the sample size needed to ensure that the results are

statistically significant. Higher confidence levels require larger samples (Andrade, 2020).

- **Anticipated Degree of Difference**: The expected effect size or degree of difference between study groups influences sample size. Smaller anticipated differences require larger samples to detect statistically significant effects (Schuster et al., 2021).

- **Population Size**: The size of the population from which the sample is drawn also impacts the sample size. Larger populations generally require larger samples to accurately represent the population (Daniel, 2012).

Importance of Larger Samples

The larger the sample, the more valid and accurate the study becomes. Larger samples are more likely to be representative of the population, reducing sampling error and increasing the generalizability of the findings (Etikan, Musa, & Alkassim, 2016).

Why Choose Bigger Samples?

Larger samples provide a more accurate reflection of the population, enhancing the reliability and validity of the study results. They reduce the margin of error and increase the power of the study, making it easier to detect significant differences or relationships (Faber & Fonseca, 2014).

When Can You Have a Small Sample?

Small samples are often used in case studies, where the focus is on in-depth analysis of a specific instance or phenomenon rather than generalizing to a larger population. Case studies provide detailed insights but are limited in their ability to generalize findings (Yin, 2018).

How to Analyze Statistics

Reliability

Reliability refers to the extent to which an experiment, measurement, or test yields the same results when repeated under identical conditions. It is a measure of consistency. For example, if a scale consistently shows the same weight for an object when measured multiple times, it is considered reliable (Creswell & Creswell, 2018).

Examples of Reliability:

- **Bathroom Scale**: A bathroom scale that shows the same weight each time a person steps on it within a short period is reliable.
- **Test-Retest Reliability**: A psychological test administered to the same group of people at two different points in time should yield similar results if it is reliable (Furr & Bacharach, 2014).

Validity

Validity is the degree to which an instrument measures what it is intended to measure. Establishing validity is more challenging than establishing reliability. An instrument that is not reliable can never be valid, but an instrument that is reliable does not necessarily have to be valid (Polit & Beck, 2017).

Examples of Validity:

- **Thermometer**: A thermometer is a valid instrument for measuring temperature but not for measuring height.
- **Content Validity**: A math test that includes questions covering all topics taught in the course has high content validity (Cohen, Manion, & Morrison, 2018).
- **Explanation**: If a thermometer is valid for measuring temperature, it is likely to be reliable because it consistently measures temperature accurately. However, if a scale is used to measure temperature, it is neither valid nor reliable for that purpose (Creswell & Creswell, 2018).

Measures of Central Tendency

The three most common measures of central tendency are the mean, median, and mode. The type and distribution of the data determine which measures of central tendency (and spread) are most appropriate (Gravetter & Wallnau, 2020).

The Mean

The mean is the sum of all scores or values divided by the total number of scores. It is also known as the average and is the most widely used measure of central tendency in statistical tests of significance. However, the mean is the most sensitive to extreme scores (Gravetter & Wallnau, 2020).

Example of Mean: If five infants had Apgar scores of 7, 8, 8, 9, and 8, you would calculate the sum of the values and divide by the total number of infants:

$$Mean = (57 + 8 + 8 + 9 + 8) \div 5 = 8$$

In the example given above, if one infant was severely depressed at the time of Apgar scoring and was given a value of 1 instead of 9, the mean would then be:

$$Mean = (57 + 8 + 8 + 1 + 8) \div 5 = 6.4$$

This demonstrates how the mean is affected by extreme values.

The Median

The median is the measure of central tendency that relates to the middle score, that is, the point on a numerical scale above and below which 50 percent of the cases fall (Field, 2018).

Example of Median: For the set of numbers 2, 2, 2, 3, **4, 5**, 6, 6, 8, 9, the median is 4.5, which is the value that divides the cases exactly in half. Since we have an even number of values, we take the average of the middle two:

$$Median = (4 + 5) \div 2 = 4.5$$

A characteristic of the median is that its calculation does not take into account the qualitative value of the individual scores. For example, in the previous sample, if the values were 2, 2, 2, 3, 4, 5, 6, 6, 8, 84, the median would still be 4.5, demonstrating its robustness to extreme values.

The Mode

The mode is the score or value that occurs most frequently in a distribution of scores (Gravetter & Wallnau, 2020).

Example of Mode: Inspect the following distribution of numbers: 30, 31, 31, 32, 33, 33, 33, 33, 34, 35, 36. The mode is 33, as it appears most frequently in the distribution.

Measures of Variability

Measures of variability should be interpreted as distances on a scale of values, unlike averages that are points representing a central value (Ciarleglio, 2020).

Types of Variability

There are four primary types of variability:

1. The range
2. Standard deviation
3. Variance
4. Inter-percentile measures

The Range

The range is the difference between the highest and lowest values in a distribution of scores (SAGE Publications, 2020). For example, if test scores for students range from 98 to 60, the range is calculated as follows:

Range=98−60=38

In research findings, the range is often reported as the maximum and minimum values without the subtracted value.

Advantages of Range:

1. It provides a quick estimate of variability.
2. It offers information about the two endpoints of the distribution.

Disadvantages of Range:

1. It is unstable since it is based only on two scores.
2. It tends to increase with sample size.
3. It is sensitive to extreme values (SpringerLink, 2020).

Standard Deviation

Standard deviation is the most frequently used statistic for measuring the degree of variability in a set of scores. It describes the average spread of scores or values around the mean and indicates how much each score is scattered from the mean (Ciarleglio, 2020).

Characteristics of Standard Deviation:

- The greater the spread of a distribution, the greater the variability, indicating a more heterogeneous group.
- The more the values cluster around the mean, the smaller the amount of variability or deviation, indicating a more homogeneous group (SAGE Publications, 2020).

Example of Standard Deviation:

If the test scores are 60, 70, 80, 90, and 100, the mean is 80. The deviations from the mean are -20, -10, 0, 10, and 20. Squaring these deviations and averaging them gives the variance, and the square root of the variance gives the standard deviation.

Normal Distribution and Frequency Distribution:

Normal Distribution

A normal distribution, often referred to as a Gaussian distribution, is a continuous probability distribution that is symmetrical around its mean, creating a bell-shaped curve. This distribution is characterized by its mean (average) and standard deviation (measure of spread). In healthcare, normal distributions are frequently used to model variables such as blood pressure, cholesterol levels, and body temperature (Limpert & Stahel, 2011).

Example: In a study measuring the blood pressure of a large population, the data might follow a normal distribution, with most individuals having blood pressure levels around the mean, and fewer individuals having extremely high or low blood pressure levels (Limpert & Stahel, 2011).

Frequency Distribution

A frequency distribution is a summary of how often different values occur within a dataset. It helps in understanding the spread and pattern of the data, making it easier to identify trends, outliers, and potential factors affecting a process (Whyte & Kelly, 2018).

Example: In a healthcare setting, a frequency distribution might be used to display the number of patients with different ranges of cholesterol levels. This can help determine if certain factors, such as diet or medication, are influencing cholesterol levels (Whyte & Kelly, 2018).

Simplified Examples in Healthcare

- **Normal Distribution Example**: The distribution of systolic blood pressure in a large sample of adults is often normally distributed. Most individuals will have blood pressure values close to the mean, with fewer individuals having very high or very low values (Limpert & Stahel, 2011).
- **Frequency Distribution Example**: A hospital might use a frequency distribution to display the number of patients admitted with different ranges of body mass index (BMI). This can help identify trends in

obesity rates and the effectiveness of weight management programs (Whyte & Kelly, 2018).

Variance

Variance measures the average degree to which each point differs from the mean. It is the square of the standard deviation and provides a mathematical expectation of the average squared deviations from the mean (SpringerLink, 2020). Variance is useful in statistical modeling and hypothesis testing.

Advantages of Variance:

1. It uses all data points, providing a comprehensive measure of variability.
2. It is essential for various statistical analyses, including ANOVA and regression.

Disadvantages of Variance:

1. It is not in the same units as the original data, making interpretation less intuitive.
2. It can be influenced by extreme values.

Example of Variance:

Using the same test scores (60, 70, 80, 90, 100), the mean is 80. The squared deviations from the mean are 400, 100, 0, 100, and 400. The average of these squared deviations is the variance, which is 200.

A break down for further clarification:

Mean:

Mean = $(60 + 70 + 80 + 90 + 100) / 5 = 80$

Squared Deviations from the mean:

* For 60: $(60 - 80)^2 = 400$

* For 70: $(70 - 80)^2 = 100$
* For 80: $(80 - 80)^2 = 0$
* For 90: $(90 - 80)^2 = 100$
* For 100: $(100 - 80)^2 = 400$

Variance:

The variance as the average of these squared deviations:

Variance = $(400 + 100 + 0 + 100 + 400) / 5 = 200$

Inter-percentile Measures

Inter-percentile measures, such as the interquartile range (IQR), describe the spread of the middle 50% of values in a distribution. The IQR is the difference between the 75th percentile (Q3) and the 25th percentile (Q1) (Bornmann & Williams, 2020).

Advantages of Inter-percentile Measures:

1. They are less affected by extreme values compared to the range.
2. They provide a clear picture of the central tendency and spread of the data.

Disadvantages of Inter-percentile Measures:

1. They do not consider all data points, potentially missing some variability.
2. They can be less informative for distributions with significant skewness.

Example of Inter-percentile Measures:

For a dataset of test scores: 55, 60, 65, 70, 75, 80, 85, 90, 95, 100, the 25th percentile (Q1) is 65, and the 75th percentile (Q3) is 90. The IQR is calculated as:

$$IQR = Q3 - Q1 = 90 - 65 = 25$$

Inter percentile clinical and quality applications:

Inter percentile measures are widely used in various fields, including health and clinical pathway development. Growth charts, for instance, are a common application of inter percentile measures. These charts often use measurements between the 25th and 75th percentiles to represent normal growth, as seen in the National Center for Health Statistics Growth Charts (Kuczmarski et al., 2000). This range helps in identifying children who are growing at a typical rate compared to their peers.

In clinical pathway development, inter percentile measures are crucial for designing effective and efficient care plans. Clinical pathways should be developed based on the interquartile range (IQR) of the designated population to ensure that the pathways are tailored to the average patient type (Rotter et al., 2010). This approach ensures that the majority of patients receive care that is appropriate for their specific needs, improving overall treatment outcomes.

Hypothesis testing:

Hypothesis testing is a fundamental aspect of statistical analysis in healthcare quality, allowing researchers to make inferences about populations based on sample data. The process involves formulating a null hypothesis (H0) and an alternative hypothesis (H1), then using statistical tests to determine whether there is enough evidence to reject the null hypothesis in favor of the alternative.

One common application of hypothesis testing in healthcare is in the evaluation of treatment effectiveness. For example, a study might test the hypothesis that a new drug is more effective than a standard treatment. The null hypothesis (H0) would state that there is no difference in effectiveness between the two treatments, while the alternative hypothesis (H1) would suggest that there is a significant difference.

In a study by Silva-Ayçaguer et al. (2010), the authors evaluated the use of null hypothesis significance testing (NHST) in health sciences research. They found that while NHST is widely used, its inferential validity has been criticized. The study highlighted the importance of not solely relying on p-values but also considering confidence intervals to provide a more comprehensive understanding of the data (Silva-Ayçaguer et al., 2010).

Another example is the use of hypothesis testing in quality improvement initiatives. For instance, a hospital might implement a new protocol to reduce patient wait times and use hypothesis testing to evaluate its effectiveness. The null hypothesis would state that the new protocol does not reduce wait times, while the alternative hypothesis would suggest that it does. By analyzing pre- and post-implementation data, researchers can determine whether the observed changes are statistically significant.

McNulty (2022) provided a logical analysis of NHST, emphasizing the need for transparency in the assumptions underlying hypothesis tests. The study discussed the common misinterpretations of p-values and the importance of understanding the limitations of NHST in making clinical decisions (McNulty, 2022).

P-value

The p-value is a fundamental concept in statistical hypothesis testing, representing the probability of obtaining test results at least as extreme as the observed results, assuming that the null hypothesis is true (Stahel, 2021). It is used to determine the statistical significance of the results of an experiment or study. A p-value less than 0.05 has traditionally been considered the threshold for statistical significance, meaning that there is less than a 5% probability that the observed results are due to chance (Ioannidis, 2019).

Historically, when the p-value is found to be less than 0.05, researchers have declared their results statistically significant and rejected the null hypothesis (Stahel, 2021). This practice has been widely adopted in various fields of research, including social sciences, medicine, and psychology. However, the reliance on a fixed threshold for significance has been criticized for oversimplifying the interpretation of statistical results and potentially leading to misleading conclusions (Ioannidis, 2019).

Recent discussions in the statistical community have highlighted the limitations of the p-value and the need for more nuanced approaches to statistical inference. For instance, the American Statistical Association (ASA) has emphasized that p-values do not measure the probability that the studied hypothesis is true or the probability that the data were produced by random chance alone (Ioannidis, 2019). Instead, p-values should be considered as one piece of evidence among many in the context of the study design, data quality, and other relevant factors.

Moreover, some researchers have proposed alternative measures to complement or replace the p-value. For example, confidence intervals provide a range of values within which the true effect size is likely to fall, offering more information about the precision and uncertainty of the estimates (Stahel, 2021). Additionally, measures such as effect sizes and Bayesian approaches have been suggested to provide a more comprehensive understanding of the results (Ioannidis, 2019).

Errors in hypothesis testing:

In hypothesis testing, two primary types of errors can occur: Type I and Type II errors. Understanding these errors is crucial for interpreting the results of statistical tests accurately.

Type I Error (False Positive)

A Type I error occurs when the null hypothesis (H0) is true, but it is incorrectly rejected. This means that the test suggests there is an effect or difference when, in reality, there is none. The probability of committing a Type I error is denoted by alpha (α), which is the significance level set by the researcher (usually 0.05).

- **Example in Healthcare:** Consider a clinical trial testing a new drug to reduce blood pressure. The null hypothesis (H0) states that the new drug has no effect on blood pressure. If the trial results in a p-value less than 0.05, the null hypothesis is rejected, suggesting the drug is effective. However, if the drug actually has no effect and the observed difference is due to random chance, this constitutes a Type I error (Silva-Ayçaguer et al., 2010).

Here is another simplified example illustrating the use of a p-value in a study:

The p-value for the ratio of missed appointment rates was less than 0.03. This result led us to conclude that there was little evidence to support the null hypothesis, which stated that men and women had the same rate of missed appointments. Consequently, we decided that men probably had a higher rate of missed appointments.

As the p-value decreases, the significance of the results increases, indicating stronger evidence against the null hypothesis.

Type II Error (False Negative)

A Type II error occurs when the null hypothesis is false, but it is not rejected. This means that the test fails to detect an effect or difference that actually exists. The probability of committing a Type II error is denoted by beta (β), and it is related to the power of the test (power = $1 - \beta$).

- **Example in Healthcare:** Imagine a study evaluating a new screening test for a disease. The null hypothesis (H0) states that the test does not detect the disease. If the test fails to identify the disease in patients who actually have it, this is a Type II error. For instance, if a new cancer screening test misses detecting cancer in patients who have it, the study has committed a Type II error (McNulty, 2022).

Balancing Type I and Type II Errors

There is a trade-off between Type I and Type II errors. Reducing the significance level (α) to minimize Type I errors increases the risk of Type II errors, and vice versa. Researchers must balance these risks based on the context and consequences of the errors.

Tests of Statistical Significance

T-Test

A t-test is a statistical test used to determine if there is a significant difference between the means of two groups. There are two main types of t-tests: independent t-tests and paired t-tests.

- **Independent t-test**: This test compares the means of two independent groups. For example, it can be used to compare the mean blood pressure levels of patients receiving two different treatments (Smith & Jones, 2020).
- **Paired t-test**: This test compares the means of two related groups. For example, it can be used to compare the mean blood pressure levels of patients before and after receiving a treatment (Smith & Jones, 2020).

In healthcare, an independent t-test might be used to compare the effectiveness of two different medications on lowering blood pressure. If the p-value obtained from the t-test is less than 0.05, it indicates that there is a statistically significant difference between the two groups (Smith & Jones, 2020).

ANOVA (Analysis of Variance)

ANOVA is used to compare the means of three or more groups to see if at least one group mean is different from the others. There are different types of ANOVA, including one-way ANOVA and two-way ANOVA.

- **One-way ANOVA**: This test is used when comparing the means of three or more independent groups based on one independent variable. For example, comparing the mean recovery times of patients using three different types of physical therapy (Brown, 2019).
- **Two-way ANOVA**: This test is used when comparing the means based on two independent variables. For example, comparing the mean recovery times of patients using three different types of physical therapy across two different age groups (Brown, 2019).

In healthcare, ANOVA can be used to compare the effectiveness of different treatments across multiple groups. If the p-value from the ANOVA is less than 0.05, it suggests that there is a significant difference among the group means (Brown, 2019).

Linear Regression

Linear regression is used to understand the relationship between a dependent variable and one independent variable. It helps in predicting the outcome of the dependent variable based on the value of the independent variable.

- **Example**: In a healthcare study, linear regression might be used to predict patient recovery time (dependent variable) based on the dosage of a medication (independent variable) (Johnson & Lee, 2021).

Linear regression is useful in healthcare for identifying trends and making predictions based on the relationship between variables (Johnson & Lee, 2021).

Multivariate Regression

Multivariate regression is used to understand the relationship between one dependent variable and two or more independent variables. This method helps in predicting the outcome of the dependent variable based on the values of the independent variables.

- **Example**: In a healthcare study, multivariate regression might be used to predict patient recovery time (dependent variable) based on age, treatment type, and initial health status (independent variables) (Johnson & Lee, 2021).

Multivariate regression is particularly useful in healthcare for adjusting for confounding variables and understanding the combined effect of multiple factors on an outcome (Johnson & Lee, 2021).

Dependent and Independent Variables

- **Dependent variable**: The outcome that is being measured in a study. For example, blood pressure levels in a study measuring the effect of a new drug.
- **Independent variable**: The variable that is being manipulated or categorized to observe its effect on the dependent variable. For example, the type of drug administered to patients (Johnson & Lee, 2021).

Simplified Examples in Healthcare

- **T-Test Example**: Comparing the mean blood pressure of patients before and after taking a new medication. If the p-value is less than 0.05, it indicates a significant difference in blood pressure levels before and after the medication (Smith & Jones, 2020).
- **ANOVA Example**: Comparing the mean recovery times of patients using three different rehabilitation programs. If the p-value is less than 0.05, it suggests that at least one rehabilitation program leads to a significantly different recovery time (Brown, 2019).
- **Linear Regression Example**: Predicting patient recovery time based on the dosage of a medication. This helps in understanding how the dosage influences recovery time (Johnson & Lee, 2021).
- **Multivariate Regression Example**: Predicting patient recovery time based on age, type of treatment, and initial health status. This helps in understanding how these factors collectively influence recovery time (Johnson & Lee, 2021).

References

1. Ackoff, R. L. (1989). From data to wisdom. Journal of Applied Systems Analysis, 16(1), 3-9.
2. Andrade, C. (2020). Sample size and its importance in research. Indian Journal of Psychological Medicine, 42(1), 102-103.
3. Babbie, E., Halley, F., & Zaino, J. (2007). Adventures in social research: Data analysis using SPSS 14.0 and 15.0 for Windows (6th ed.). SAGE Publications.
4. Baker, R., Brick, J. M., Bates, N. A., Battaglia, M., Couper, M. P., Dever, J. A., ... & Tourangeau, R. (2013). Summary report of the AAPOR task force on non-probability sampling. Journal of Survey Statistics and Methodology, 1(2), 90-143.
5. Bornmann, L., & Williams, R. (2020). An evaluation of percentile measures of citation impact, and a proposal for making them better. Scientometrics, 124, 1457-1478. https://doi.org/10.1007/s11192-020-03512-7
6. Bornstein, M. H., Jager, J., & Putnick, D. L. (2013). Sampling in developmental science: Situations, shortcomings, solutions, and standards. Developmental Review, 33(4), 357-370.
7. Brown, A. (2019). Statistical methods in healthcare research. New York, NY: Health Press.
8. Ciarleglio, A. (2020). Measures of variability and precision in statistics: appreciating, untangling and applying concepts. BJPsych Advances, 27(2), 137-139. https://doi.org/10.1192/bja.2020.41
9. Cohen, L., Manion, L., & Morrison, K. (2018). Research methods in education (8th ed.). Routledge.
10. Creswell, J. W., & Creswell, J. D. (2018). Research design: Qualitative, quantitative, and mixed methods approaches (5th ed.). SAGE Publications.
11. Daniel, J. (2012). Sampling essentials: Practical guidelines for making sampling choices. SAGE Publications.
12. Davenport, T. H., & Prusak, L. (1998). Working knowledge: How organizations manage what they know. Harvard Business Press.
13. Etikan, I., Musa, S. A., & Alkassim, R. S. (2016). Comparison of convenience sampling and purposive sampling. American Journal of Theoretical and Applied Statistics, 5(1), 1-4.
14. Faber, J., & Fonseca, L. M. (2014). How sample size influences research outcomes. Dental Press Journal of Orthodontics, 19(4), 27-29.

15. Field, A. (2018). Discovering statistics using IBM SPSS statistics (5th ed.). SAGE Publications.

16. Furr, R. M., & Bacharach, V. R. (2014). Psychometrics: An introduction (2nd ed.). SAGE Publications.

17. Gravetter, F. J., & Wallnau, L. B. (2020). Statistics for the behavioral sciences (10th ed.). Cengage Learning.

18. Ioannidis, J. P. A. (2019). Publishing research with P-values: Prescribe more stringent statistical significance or proscribe statistical significance? European Heart Journal, 40(31), 2553-2554. https://doi.org/10.1093/eurheartj/ehz555

19. Johnson, R., & Lee, M. (2021). Advanced statistics for health sciences. Boston, MA: Medical Publishers.

20. . Kadam, P., & Bhalerao, S. (2010). Sample size calculation. International Journal of Ayurveda Research, 1(1), 55-57.

21. Katz, M. H. (2006). Multivariable analysis: A practical guide for clinicians. Cambridge University Press.

22. Kuczmarski, R. J., Ogden, C. L., Guo, S. S., Grummer-Strawn, L. M., Flegal, K. M., Mei, Z., ... & Johnson, C. L. (2000). CDC growth charts for the United States: methods and development. Vital and health statistics. Series 11, Data from the national health survey, (246), 1-190.

23. Lewis-Beck, M., Bryman, A., & Liao, T. F. (Eds.). (2004). The SAGE encyclopedia of social science research methods (Vol. 1). SAGE Publications.

24. Limpert, E., & Stahel, W. A. (2011). Problems with using the normal distribution – and ways to improve quality and efficiency of data analysis. PLOS ONE, 6(7), e21403. https://doi.org/10.1371/journal.pone.0021403

25. McNulty, R. (2022). A logical analysis of null hypothesis significance testing using popular terminology. BMC Medical Research Methodology, 22(1), 244.

26. Naderifar, M., Goli, H., & Ghaljaie, F. (2017). Snowball sampling: A purposeful method of sampling in qualitative research. Strides in Development of Medical Education, 14(3), e67670.

27. Nonaka, I., & Takeuchi, H. (1995). The knowledge-creating company: How Japanese companies create the dynamics of innovation. Oxford University Press.

28. Polit, D. F., & Beck, C. T. (2017). Nursing research: Generating and assessing evidence for nursing practice (10th ed.). Wolters Kluwer.

29. Rotter, T., Kinsman, L., James, E., Machotta, A., Willis, J., Snow, P., & Kugler, J. (2010). Clinical pathways: effects on professional practice, patient outcomes, length of stay, and hospital costs. Cochrane Database of Systematic Reviews, (3).

30. Rowley, J. (2007). The wisdom hierarchy: Representations of the DIKW hierarchy. Journal of Information Science, 33(2), 163-180.

31. SAGE Publications. (2020). Measures of variability. In Research Methods in Psychology. https://us.sagepub.com/sites/default/files/upm-binaries/23689_Chapter_5___Measures_of_Variability.pdf

32. Schuster, R., Kaiser, T., Terhorst, Y., Messner, E. M., Strohmeier, L.-M., & Laireiter, A.-R. (2021). Sample size planning and the impact of study context: Systematic review and recommendations by the example of psychological depression treatment. Psychological Medicine, 51(6), 902-908.

33. Silva-Ayçaguer, L. C., Suárez-Gil, P., & Fernández-Somoano, A. (2010). The null hypothesis significance test in health sciences research (1995-2006): Statistical analysis and interpretation. BMC Medical Research Methodology, 10(1), 44.

34. Smith, T., & Jones, L. (2020). Introduction to biostatistics. Chicago, IL: Science Press.

35. Springfield, L. (2020). Measures of variability. In Statistical Methods for Psychology. https://link.springer.com/chapter/10.1007/978-1-4612-4000-6_4

36. Stahel, W. A. (2021). New relevance and significance measures to replace p-values. PLOS ONE, 16(6), e0252991. https://doi.org/10.1371/journal.pone.0252991

37. Stevens, S. S. (1946). On the theory of scales of measurement. Science, 103(2684), 677-680.

38. Velleman, P. F., & Wilkinson, L. (1993). Nominal, ordinal, interval, and ratio typologies are misleading. The American Statistician, 47(1), 65-72.

39. Whyte, M. B., & Kelly, P. (2018). The normal range: it is not normal and it is not a range. Postgraduate Medical Journal, 94(1117), 613-616. https://doi.org/10.1136/postgradmedj-2018-135983

40. Yin, R. K. (2018). Case study research and applications: Design and methods (6th ed.). SAGE Publications.

Chapter 10

Change Management and Process Improvement Methods

Change in healthcare organizations could be planned or unplanned for, and could be either in structure, processes, which leads definitely to change in outcomes. Decades ago in farming, heavy machinery reduced the number of hands needed to reap the harvest making it an easier, faster, and more efficient process. The application of new technologies in healthcare changed the way medicine is practiced today. Who would of imagined open heart surgeries would be less in numbers with the introduction of new non-invasive catheterization techniques, or the application of electronic medical records, making it faster and easier for the healthcare provider and caregiver to access his or her patient's records at a click of a button, and tying its implementation to reimbursement in some healthcare systems, pushing for its adaptation and change.

Change today or fade away

In the examples given above, a farmer that did not adapt to the changes in farming, grazing, and hasting would of ran out of business by hiring more workers and by harvesting less. Healthcare organizations and hospitals in the United States that do not implement electronic health records are losing reimbursement from the largest single payer in the nation the Centers of Medicare and Medicaid. Some photography and film developing companies are out of business today with the introduction of digital and instant photography. The message is clear, the whole world is changing, and those who fail to improve, adapt, or change will definitely find themselves as a result out of business, since it is inevitable and also an essential pillar of growth.

Reasons employees and organizations resist change

Insecurity: People derive security from doing the same things the same way, and any changes are considered a threat. Insecurity could be either **economic**; such as losing the job, thus a reduction in pay, or **social;** such as being distant from the coworkers that bonds have developed over a previous part of time.

Habitual challenge: A job with time becomes easy to perform as habits and skills develop. Change causes an interruption of that easiness, which causes fear of difficulty learning how to perform on a new job.

Organizational and work group inertia: Organizations promote stability, as they carefully select employees and train them to perform either alone or in groups for certain jobs, which cause forces of resistance to accept change.

Unsuccessful previous change experiences: As it implies *"Once bitten twice shy"* an organization or a person who has failed a previous experience in anything and/or change are reluctant to endure another attempt. (Greenberg & Baron, 2008)

Change Models in Theory

Lewin's Change Model

Kurt Lewin proposed that for change to occur driving forces must be greater than restraining forces and thus the greater the driving forces the faster the change. Motives of change could be frustration and/or dissatisfaction with the status quo, which creates an urge to change.

Lewin summarizes the change process into three stages:

1. *Unfreezing:* The recognition of need to change or a sense of urgency, as the current state is undesirable or dangerous to stay in, such as a financial loss or a threat.
2. *Intervening change:* In this stage a change actually occurs with restructuring and creating a desirable state.
3. *Refreeze:* Refreezing occurs when the new state of changes become habitual as the changes are incorporated as they freeze again and become the new culture or practice. (Levasseur, 2001)

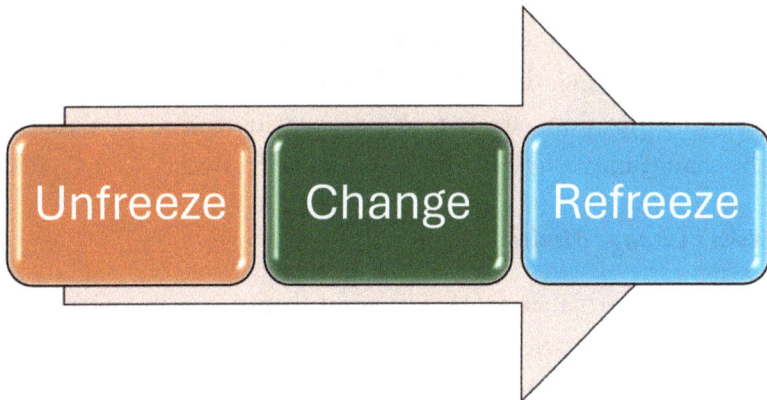

Figure 10.1 : Summary of Lewin's Change Model

DeWeaver and Gillespie's Change Model

The Stages of this change model are broken down into 5 stages as described by (DeWeaver & Gillespie, 1997) and are as following:

First Stage- *Awareness*: The individual is aware of a change plan, but does not have an opinion towards it and even is in denial at this stage. This happens when an advertisement of a change is announced to increase awareness in an organization.

Second stage- *Curiosity*: As it implies the individual is concerned and becomes curious by inquiring about the effect of change. The organization is obliged to explain clearly and acknowledge the difficulties change might cause. This stage creates a level of dissatisfaction with the current state to generate interest into the newer state the organization is headed to.

Third stage- *Visualization:* The individual seeks to understand the effect of change on them along with the organization. Organization's leadership trying to change is recommended to give employees the opportunity to try the change before it is put into place.

Fourth stage- *Learning:* The individual takes part in learning how to implement the change and could share any suggestions or ideas to the change. Organizations in this stage are supposedly educating and training staff at this level.

Fifth stage- *Use:* The individual uses the change actively and becomes accustomed to it in their daily work. He or she is able to explain the change to others. Organizations are required to provide technical assistance to make the change move rapidly, efficiently, and effectively.

Prochaska's Change Model

James Prochaska's explanation of behavioral change is useful when working with staff members, patients, and/or providers. The model explains the individual preparedness to change his or her behavior rather than changes in organizational processes. Prochaska summarized the change of behavior in six steps as following:

- Precontemplation: The individual has no intention to change practices or behaviors within the next six months
- Contemplation: The individual at this stage has the intention to change practices or behaviors with the next six months.
- Action: The individual has changed the intended behavior for less than six months.
- Maintenance: The individual has changed the behavior for more than six months.
- Termination: The previous behavior will never return as it is terminated and the individual is able to cope without fear to go back. (Prochaska & DiClemente, 2005)

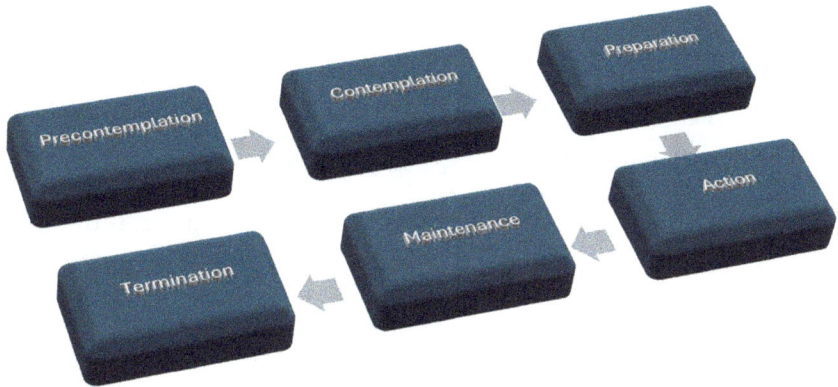

Figure 10.2: Prochaska's stages in behavioral change

Kotter's Change Model

John Kotter suggests and associates emotional feelings and the heart with change. He describes an eight step change model as following:

Step 1: Elevate urgency: The most critical to Kotter is to create a feeling of urgency with evidence that change is required.

Step 2: Guiding team build up: Influential leaders are employed at this stage to promote for change. Picking the proper and committed people is extremely important and vital for the success of the change efforts.

Step 3: Get the vision right: A clear vision is always essential. Leadership is responsible for proper direction, which will steer into the new changing direction.

Step 4: Communicate: Once a vision and strategy have been produced, the organization is required to communicate, communicate, communicate! This step must be repeated throughout the change effort and the message must be direct, simple, and concise.

Step 5: Empower action: Barriers and obstacles must be removed along with promoting confidence in change by giving the employees the ability to act.

Step 6: Create short term wins: The creation of short term wins inspires and energizes users of the change.

Step 7: Do not let up: The change process is not over until change is a reality and fully implemented. Leaders are supposed to build on short term wins and keeping the urgency alive.

Step 8: Make change stick: This is the most difficult step as it is the end of the change process as it is tough to sustain and ingrain. (Kotter & Cohen, 2002)

Importance of Process Improvement in Healthcare

With the emerging concerns of the inflation in the healthcare cost, placing the industry under increased scrutiny. The Institute of Medicine's (IOM) report in 1999 titled *To Err is Human*, answered and documented the alarming status of the U.S. Healthcare system by defining some of its shortcomings.

According to the report almost all of medical errors that occur in healthcare organizations today are a result of faulty processes and systems. The blame is not fully placed on the healthcare providers. The variability of processes in healthcare along with a plethora of contributing factors such as provider's educational background and experience along with different case mix and the biology all add to healthcare's complexity. Due to these factors, it is highly vital to embrace process improvement (PI) techniques to define the shortcomings and deficiencies in the system, and work on preventing these errors from happening again.

Most accrediting bodies such as the Joint Commission in the United States (TJC, 2024), and the Joint Commission International (JCI, 2024), and the Central Board for Accreditation of Healthcare Institutions (CBAHI, 2024) as examples of bodies that require healthcare organizations to show evidence of continuous process improvement projects throughout their departments as a standard of quality and excellence.

In our daily lives, we come across process improvements without training. In example if we dial the wrong phone number using a landline telephone, we concentrate the second time dialing the number slowly and get the correct number by proof dialing, which is a process improvement that leads to better outcomes. We will introduce in detail several process improvement techniques in the following section.

Process Improvement techniques

There are many process improvement techniques and tools used in healthcare to assist an organization to assess for change. It is important to know that "All changes do not necessarily lead to improvement, but all improvement requires change" (IHI, 2014).

Plan-Do-Check-Act (PDCA)

Also known as Plan-Do-Study-Act (PDSA) and Plan-Do-Check-Adjust

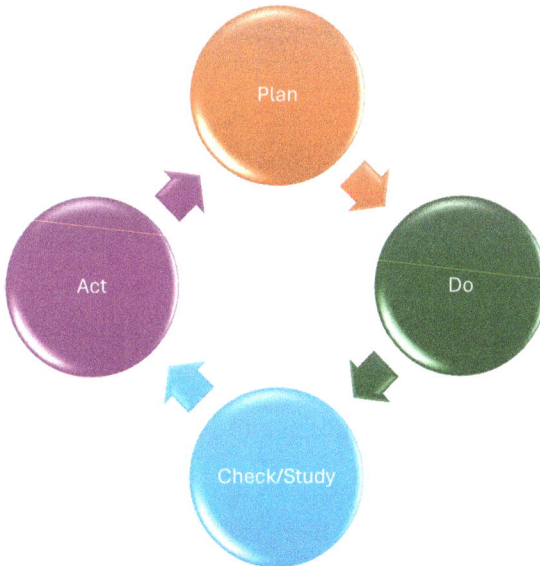

Figure 10.3: PDCA/PDSA Continuous Process Improvement Cycle

Are both a four step cycle in management for control and continuous improvement of processes and outcomes. This basic concept we practice daily when we plan to wake up at a certain time and do our alarm watches and check if we set the correct time and act to wake up when the alarm rings in the morning. PDCA was the precursor to PDSA as it was introduced by the American engineer/statistician Walter Andrew Shewhart, and is also known to be the Shewhart wheel. This same cycle was amended by W. Edward Deming, also an engineer/statistician as he substituted the "C" to "S" and coined the PDSA cycle or the Deming cycle. The PDCA/PDSA is the most acceptable and widely used technique in healthcare, due to its simplicity and

- **P-*Plan:*** The Plan stage of the PDSA or PDCA cycle is important, since any move needs a plan. It sets out the guidelines for the whole process, which includes the outcome expectations along with the objectives and goals.
- **D-*Do:*** Actual implementation of the plan occurs in this stage, such as data collection. Along with collecting the relevant measurement data or metrics.
- **C/S-*Check / Study:*** This stage of the cycle involves studying and checking the results obtained and collected in the "DO" step, hunting for deviations from the expected.
- **A-*Act:*** In this last step of the PDSA/PDCA cycle, it is necessary to define and act upon corrective actions on areas where there are significant differences between actual and planned results. It is important to analyze the results to determine the root causes wherever possible. Once this has been achieved, it is possible to implement the process improvement changes (Chiarini, 2011).

The PDSA / PDCA cycle is repetitive. So, once it has competed, it is necessary to return to the beginning and see what further improvements could be made.

A simple project example of a PDCA/PDSA cycle in healthcare would be as following:

PLAN: A hospital begins to realize that the length of stay (LOS) at the emergency department is too high, and they plan to perform a PDCA project to find a solution and improve the LOS.

Using some of the quality improvement tools that are outlined in the following chapter, such as visualizing the whole patient experience in a process map, a Root Cause Analysis (RCA). The PI team then pinpoints the cause of the elongated length of stay at the ED, and defines a goal of time reduction and by a certain time, which usually does not exceed three to six months.

DO: In this step of the cycle the PI project team members would meet and brainstorm (Explained in detail in the chapter Quality Improvement tools and Methods). After brainstorming, The PI team would have an action plan for this PI project as they would realize the gap areas and will assign areas of improvement to specific team members.

CHECK/STUDY: The team would check or study the results of waiting times at the baseline and current and compare to identify improvements. Updating the action plan usually happens at this step.

ACT: At this stage if the waiting times are not improving as planned, as there is still room for improvement, and reassessment of the action plan after adjustment. If the goals were achieved then it is time to standardize and act upon the new standardization, in addition to expand this practice to other departments if applicable or appropriate.

FOCUS PDCA

Dr. Paul Batalden formed the Quality Resource Group (QRG) in the 1980's, which is part of the Hospital Corporation of America (HCA). QRG developed this new process improvement model and named it FOCUS-PDCA. The model name is an acronym that describes the basic components of the improvement process. The steps include added to the above mentioned PDCA steps as they precede them:

F- Find a process to improve:

- o Define the process
- o Identify the customer/s and who will benefit from this improvement

O-Organize an effort to work on improvement:

- o Choose people who are involved and experienced in the process to be improved
- o A team with an appropriate number of members that represents multi levels of the organization
- o A methodology must be developed to document the progress of the project.

C-Clarify current knowledge of the process:

- o A revision of the current state of the process
- o Outline and analyze the process and compare expected and actual performance

U-Understand process variation and causes of this variation:

- o Learn the causes of variation by measuring the process using performance indicators.
- o Pick measurable and controllable variables.

S-Select a strategy for continued improvement:

- o Identification of the actionable improvement to the process
- o Support the proposed action with evidence that is documented

(Batalden, 1992)

The FOCUS steps are followed by the PDCA/PDSA cycle mentioned in the previous section.

Kaizen

Kaizen is the Japanese word for "improvement", where "Kai" means change and "Zen" means good. It is the involvement of everybody in ongoing and continuous improvement, including the CEO, all managers, and workers. The primary goal of a Kaizen is to eliminate waste. Kaizen started in Japanese factories post world war II, as a process improvement method to restore Japan and its manufacturing. In case of any minor anomalies in the factory all assembly line workers would stop and start a Kaizen immediately to resolve the problem. A kaizen team could be comprised of one member or more, which proves its simplicity as it is not a pre-planned project in most cases. Kaizen could be a preliminary step before a Lean or six sigma project, as the problem need to be solved is identified in this simple step. Kaizen evolved to the Toyota way. (Imai, 1997)

An example of a Kaizen small project in healthcare witnessed, Pediatric patients at a children's clinic would not sit still or began to cry and shout during ultrasound procedures. The excessive recurrence of this specific event caused frustration to both technicians at that pediatric department along with the kids' parents. The head of the department formed a Kaizen and brainstormed for an easy and innovative solution. The team reached consensus to have bubble bottles prepared at all times and blow some bubbles for this group of patients, which is certainly entertaining to everybody including the kids and children.

Ernst and Young Seven-Step "IMPROVE" Model:

Ernst and Young (EY), is a multinational consulting firm headquartered in London, England. It is considered one of the "Big four" audit groups along with the American giant Deloitte, the British PricewaterhouseCoopers, and the Dutch KPMG.

EY developed the following seven step process improvement model:

I- Identify:

- o The Problem to be addressed is identified and determined in this step.
- o The current performance level is assessed and understood.

M-Measure:

- o The extent and level of the stated problem is measured at this stage.
- o The impact on both external and internal customers is measured using available data.

P-Prioritize:

- o The possible causations are identified and listed
- o The listed causes are prioritized

R- Research:

- o The root cause is analyzed and understood.
- o In depth assessment of the root causes is done at this stage.

V-Validation:

- o Validation of the previous steps are done at this stage
- o An established monitoring system determines the effectiveness of the solutions proposed

E-Execute:

- o Solutions and standards are fully implemented and are of common practice
- o A continuation of the monitoring to assure sustenance and problem resolution

(Schiller, Miller-Kovach, & Miller, 1994).

The EY seven-step IMPROVE model specifically, is not widely used in healthcare, although the concepts are of similar practice.

The "FADE" cycle Model:

The American based healthcare quality consulting firm Organizational Development (ODI) developed a four step process improvement model and named it the "FADE" cycle (Brown, 2008), and is broken down as following:

F- Focus:

- o A problem is identified, selected, and verified based on primary data. A problem statement is written.

A- Analyze:

- o   The problem is analyzed by data collection and creating a baseline to understand the problem in detail.

D- Develop:

- o   A plan for improvement is developed to be implemented with a promising solution/s

E- Execute:

- o   The plan at this stage is executed, and the impact is monitored and recorded for proof of sustenance. (Milakovich, 1995)

The Lean Enterprise model:

Lean thinking coined by James Womack the MIT professor, and also called lean manufacturing or the TOYOTA methodology as it evolved from the automobile manufacturing industry in Japan (Graban, 2011). The Toyota production system's methodology main focus is to remove and eliminate waste. The common measure in lean is the touch time, which is defined as the total time a product or service is spent on by the worker, and thus the focus is emphasized on flow, and the reduction of waste. Lean is a widely accepted methodology nowadays in healthcare, since the application of statistics is lesser than six sigma. Six sigma is a better methodology that deals with widgets and is widely used in the manufacturing arena, however lean simplifies processes and eliminates waste, overcomplicated processes, workarounds, and rework in these processes, leading to the reduction of time in these processes, and thus leading us to a uniform output, reduced inventory, and a lesser variation in the processes performed. Lean is distinct from the remaining process improvement methods in that it emphasizes the investigation of getting things done efficiently along with total redesign rather than change (Womack & Jones, 2010).

Anything in excess of value is considered to be waste. The customer defines what is valued and what is not valued. Waste is any activity that does not add value to the process. The lean enterprise categorizes "Muda", which is waste into the following "TIM-WOOD":

1. **Overproduction**: It is the excessive production for the client, such as delaying patient discharges in hospitals or over producing meals that patients do not eat.
2. **Over processing:** Excessive services for the client, such as ordering too many diagnostic tests that are unnecessary. Or performing a surgical procedure when an alternative non-invasive intervention is applicable.
3. **Unnecessary Motion:** As it implies wasted movement in a working center, such as caregivers walking long distances to get or search for supplies or a medication.
4. **Unnecessary Transport**: It is the unnecessary transportation of materials and patients throughout the healthcare facility, such as patient transportation from a department to another or the transportation of goods such as meals or specimens throughout the healthcare organization.
5. **Excessive Waiting:** Timeliness is very important in healthcare. Long lines to see a caregiver or an examination room is considered to be wasteful.
6. **Defects:** Which are errors mistakes, wrong medication prescriptions.
7. **Inventory inefficiency:** It is the over stocking of unnecessary medications, supplies, or equipment until they expire or become invalid for usage. (Liker, 2003).

Six sigma 6 σ:

Six sigma is a business strategy and a process improvement methodology used in many services and in manufacturing that was developed by the U.S. phone manufacturer Motorola in 1987 (Snee, 2004). The American giant General Electric (GE), successfully implemented six sigma to reduce errors and to profit significantly (Eckes, 2002). Six sigma's goal and concept is the elimination of defects in processes, services, and eventually products to as minimum as Crosby's "zero defects". The statistical explanation of six sigma is calculated as 3.4 defects or errors in a "six digit" million opportunities (DPMO). A defect is the outcome that does not meet the specification or expectations of the customer. Any of the seven wastes mentioned in the previous section is considered a defect. As mentioned previously, Lean and six sigma are used widely nowadays in healthcare. More than of the titles and abstracts published in quality healthcare improvement literature had both of these terms stated (Walshe, 2009).

To understand the meaning of six sigma, the following table 1 as it shows a decrease in DPMO with an increase in the sigma level.

Table 10.1: Sigma (σ) value and the DPMO associated with it.

Sigma Level σ	Defects per million (DPMO)
1 σ	700,000
2 σ	308,537
3 σ	66,807
4 σ	6210
5 σ	233
6 σ	3.14

(Brown, 2008).

From the above table it is obvious that healthcare has not even reached a 4 σ level yet, since the healthcare error rate in the U.S. is about 6.2 DPMO, which is approximately 3.8 σ and about 1 σ when it comes to other activities in the healthcare sector. The six sigma methodology is still in its infancy stages when it comes to healthcare. Healthcare providers strive to reach a 5 or 6 σ level such as banking and the aviation industries. Most six sigma practitioners find healthcare and the services industry potential and fertile grounds for improvement. Six sigma methodology works well where there are high production rates of the same parts in areas such as the clinical laboratories, billing, and emergency departments (Trusko, Pexton, Gupta, & Harrington, 2007).

Six Sigma Project Outline

Six sigma's projects include five steps: define, measure, analyze, improve, and control- known as DMAIC. The DMAIC process is divided into two main themes or parts the first is familiarizing ourselves with the problem and understanding it and consists of the first three steps of the DMAIC process: Define, Measure, Analyze. The second part is the solution of the problem part, which includes the remaining two steps the improve and the control steps. The DMAIC process activities are summarized as following:

Define:

- o Defining the problem based on data.
- o Mapping of the process.

Measure:

- o The development of input, process, and output measures.
- o Baseline data is collected.
- o Flowchart process in detail to understand the current process

Analyze:

- o The analysis of root or potential causes of the defects.
- o The confirmation of the causes with supportive data.

Improve:

- o The creation of solutions for the root causes.
- o The development of plans.
- o Piloting the developed plans.
- o The actual implementation of the plans.
- o The measurement of the results.
- o The determination of the unit cost savings.

Control:

- o The standardization of the new processes.
- o The development of the monitoring systems.
- o Sustainment, communicating learned lessons, and recommendation of future improvement plans.

(Shankar, 2009).

Differences and similarities between six sigma and lean methodologies:

Both six sigma and lean management use quality management statistical tools, which are explained in detail in the quality improvement: tools and methods chapter of this textbook.

Six sigma and lean methods have a lot in common, as they use similar statistical tools, but the differences between them could be summarized as following:

- Lean primarily has been thought of as "thinking and or principles", on the contrary six sigma is considered to be a "philosophy or a standard of excellence".
- Lean is a precursor to six sigma, since it provides tools to sustain six sigma much better, whereas six sigma can be achieved without lean, but could build on lean operations.
- Lean is directed by middle management, however six sigma is driven by leadership.
- Lean impacts selected processes for speed and value, but six sigma impacts both products and processes.
- Lean is efficient; on the contrary six sigma is effective.
- Lean reduces wasted activities, and six sigma reduces waste in activities.

(Trusko, Pexton, Gupta, & Harrington, 2007).

In a nutshell, the implementation of lean would result in your meal arriving at your table faster (efficiently), but six sigma has your meal arrive to your table at a decent time, but warmer (effectively).

References:

1. Batalden, P. B. (1992). Building knowledge for improvement-an introductory guide to the use of FOCUS-PDCA. Quality Resource Group, Hospital Corporation of America. Nashville, TN.

2. Brown, J. (2008). The health care quality handbook: A professional resource and study guide. Pasadena, CA: JB Quality Solutions.

3. Central Board of Accreditation for Healthcare Institutions. (2024). Hospital Accreditation Standards Manual for Hospitals: The Official Handbook: CBAHI.

4. Chiarini, A. (2011). Japanese total quality control, TQM, Deming's system of profound knowledge, BPR, lean and Six Sigma: comparison and discussion. International Journal of Lean Six Sigma, 2(4), 332-355.

5. DeWeaver, M. F., & Gillespie, L. (1997). Real-world project management: New approaches for adapting to change and uncertainty. New York: Quality Resources.

6. Eckes, G. (2002). The Six Sigma revolution: How General Electric and others turned process into profits. Hoboken, NJ: John Wiley & Sons.

7. Graban, M. (2011). Lean Hospitals: improving quality, patient safety, and employee engagement. Boca Raton, FL: CRC Press.

8. Greenberg, J., & Baron, R. A. (2008). Behavior in organizations. New Jersey: Pearson Prentice Hall.

9. Imai, M. (1997). Gemba Kaizen: A Commonsense, Low-Cost Approach To Management. McGraw-Hill.

10. Institute for Healthcare Improvement. How to improve. Improvement methods. Retrieved from , http://www.who.int/patientsafety/education/curriculum/who_mc_topic-7.pdf

11. Joint Commission International. (2024). Joint Commission International Accreditation Standards for Hospitals. Oakbrook, IL: Joint Commission on Accreditation of Health care Organizations.

12. Joint Commission on Accreditation of Healthcare Organizations. (2024). Comprehensive Accreditation Manual for Hospitals: The Official Handbook: Camh. Joint Commission Resources.

13. Kohn, L. T., Corrigan, J. M., & Donaldson, M. S. (Eds.). (2000). To Err Is Human: Building a Safer Health System (Vol. 627). National Academies Press.

14. Kotter, J. P., & Cohen, D. S. (2002). The heart of change: Real-life stories of how people change their organizations. Boston, MA: Harvard Business Press.

15. Levasseur, R. E. (2001). People skills: Change management tools—Lewin's change model. Interfaces, 31(4), 71-73.

16. Liker, J. K. (2003). The Toyota way. New York, NY: McGraw Hill.

17. Milakovich, M. (1995). Improving service quality: achieving high performance in the public and private sectors. CRC Press.

18. Prochaska, J. O., & DiClemente, C. C. (2005). The transtheoretical approach. Handbook of psychotherapy integration.

19. Schiller, M. R., Miller-Kovach, K., & Miller, M. A. (1994). Total quality management for hospital nutrition services. Sudbury, MA: Jones & Bartlett Learning.

20. Shankar, R. (2009). Process Improvement Using Six Sigma: A DMAIC Guide. ASQ Quality Press.

21. Snee, R. D. (2004). Six–Sigma: the evolution of 100 years of business improvement methodology. International Journal of Six Sigma and Competitive Advantage, 1(1), 4-20.

22. Trusko, B. E., Pexton, C., Gupta, P. K., & Harrington, J. (2007). Improving healthcare quality and cost with Six Sigma. Upper Saddle River, NJ: Pearson Education.

23. Walshe, K. (2009). Pseudoinnovation: the development and spread of healthcare quality improvement methodologies. International Journal for Quality in Health Care.

24. Womack, J. P., & Jones, D. T. (2010). Lean thinking: banish waste and create wealth in your corporation. New York, NY: Simon and Schuster.

Chapter 11

Team Management

Understanding Working Teams

Definition of a Team

A team can be defined in various contexts, each emphasizing different aspects of collaboration and collective effort. According to Kozlowski and Ilgen (2006), a team is a group of individuals who are interdependent in their tasks, share responsibilities for outcomes, and see themselves and are seen by others as an intact social entity embedded in one or more larger social systems (Kozlowski & Ilgen, 2006).

Definition of a Working Team

A working team is a specific type of team characterized by common objectives, willingness to work together, selection and training to perform defined tasks, and interdependence among members. This concept is supported by research in organizational behavior and psychology, which emphasizes the importance of interdependence and shared goals in team settings (Hackman & Wageman, 2005).

Differences Between Teams and Groups

Teams and groups differ in several key aspects:

- **Longevity**: Teams tend to stay together longer than groups.
- **Objectives**: Teams have common objectives, whereas groups may not.

- **Interdependence**: Teams depend on one another, while most non-team groups are not interdependent.
- **Selection and Willingness**: Team members are selected and willing to work together, which is not always the case in groups (Bell et al., 2011).

Characteristics of Team Members

Team members generally:

- Have common objectives.
- Are dependent on one another in some way.
- Are willing to work together.
- Go through a selection process.
- Think of themselves as a team.

These characteristics are crucial for the functioning and success of teams. Research indicates that teams with clear goals, well-defined roles, and mutual dependence tend to perform better and achieve higher levels of satisfaction (Bell et al., 2011).

Examples of Groups

Examples of groups include a group of nurses working on a ward or a group of stewards and stewardesses working for an airline. While these individuals may work in the same environment, they do not necessarily work together in an interdependent manner, which distinguishes them from teams (National Research Council, 2015).

Scientific Insights on Teams

Team Dynamics and Effectiveness

Team dynamics and effectiveness are influenced by various factors, including team composition, task design, and the external environment. Effective teams exhibit high levels of cohesion, clear communication, and well-defined roles and responsibilities (Kozlowski & Ilgen, 2006).

Team Science

Team science involves collaborative research efforts that bring together diverse expertise to tackle complex scientific problems. Enhancing the effectiveness of team science requires understanding how teams organize, communicate, and conduct research. Factors such as team dynamics, leadership, and institutional support are crucial for the success of scientific teams (National Research Council, 2015).

Team Composition

The composition of a team significantly affects its performance. Teams with diverse skill sets and perspectives are often more innovative and effective. However, diversity can also lead to conflicts if not managed properly. Research suggests that team diversity, when coupled with inclusive practices, enhances team performance by bringing in varied viewpoints and problem-solving approaches (Bell et al., 2011).

Leadership in Teams

Leadership is a critical component of team success. Effective team leaders facilitate communication, resolve conflicts, and motivate team members. Leaders who adopt a transformational leadership style—characterized by inspiring and motivating team members—tend to foster higher levels of team performance and satisfaction (Hackman & Wageman, 2005).

Institutional Support

Institutional structures and policies also impact team effectiveness. Supportive environments that provide resources, training, and recognition for team efforts are essential. Policies that recognize and reward collaborative efforts are important for promoting effective team science (National Academies of Sciences, Engineering, and Medicine, 2015).

Types of Teams

Teams can vary widely based on several factors:

- **Supervision**: Teams can operate with or without direct supervision. Self-managed teams, for example, are given the autonomy to make decisions and manage their own activities (Cohen & Bailey, 1997).
- **Skill Composition**: Teams can be single-skilled, where all members have similar expertise, or multi-skilled, where members bring diverse skills to the table. Multi-skilled teams are often more innovative and adaptable (Edmondson & Nembhard, 2009).
- **Duration**: Teams can be formed for short-term projects or long-term objectives. Temporary teams, such as project teams, disband after achieving their goals, while permanent teams, like departmental teams, continue to work together indefinitely (Mathieu, Maynard, Rapp, & Gilson, 2008).
- **Location**: Teams can be co-located, working in the same physical space, or dispersed, working remotely across different locations. Virtual teams, which rely on digital communication tools, are increasingly common in today's globalized work environment (Gibson & Cohen, 2003).
- **Tasks**: Teams can be tasked with a single objective or multiple goals. Task complexity and variety can influence team dynamics and performance (Hackman, 2002).
- **Size**: Teams can vary in size, from small teams of three or four members to large teams of twenty or more. Smaller teams often require less supervision and can be more agile, while larger teams may benefit from a broader range of skills and perspectives but can face challenges in coordination and communication (Wheelan, 2009).

Team Size and Effects

The size of a team significantly impacts its dynamics and effectiveness. Small teams, typically consisting of three to four members, often require minimal supervision and can make decisions quickly. They benefit from close-knit relationships and clear communication channels. In contrast, larger teams, such as those with twenty or thirty members, may experience more complex interactions and require more structured management to maintain cohesion and productivity (Wheelan, 2009).

Organizational Effects on Teams

The organizational context can greatly influence team performance. Differences in objectives, approaches to tasks, and attitudes towards external stakeholders can shape how teams function. Organizational culture, policies, and support systems play crucial roles in enabling or hindering team effectiveness (Kozlowski & Ilgen, 2006).

Team Background Effects

The background and formation of a team can affect its initial performance and cohesion. Newly formed teams may face uncertainties regarding member relationships and clarity of goals. Effective onboarding and team-building activities can help mitigate these challenges and foster a sense of purpose and unity among team members (Tuckman, 1965).

Technology's Effect on Teams

Automated Factories vs. Craftsmanship

In automated factories, the primary focus is on the volume of output and consistency of the product. Teams in such environments often do not see the final product, which can impact their sense of accomplishment and connection to the work. This contrasts sharply with craftsmanship, where the quality of a single product is paramount. Craftspersons often take pride in their work, leading to higher job satisfaction and a stronger sense of individual accomplishment. The emphasis on quality over quantity allows for more personal investment in the work (Kozlowski & Ilgen, 2006).

Impact of Technology on Team Dynamics

Technology significantly shapes team dynamics and effectiveness. Digital communication tools, such as Slack and Microsoft Teams, facilitate collaboration by enabling real-time communication and information sharing, regardless of geographical location. These tools can enhance team cohesion and productivity by providing platforms for synchronous and asynchronous interactions (Gibson & Cohen, 2003). However, the reliance on technology can also introduce challenges, such as difficulties in building trust and managing conflicts in virtual teams (Morrison-Smith & Ruiz, 2020).

Benefits of Being in a Group

Being part of a group offers several psychological and social benefits:

- **Companionship**: Groups provide social interaction and companionship, which can reduce feelings of isolation and loneliness (Baumeister & Leary, 1995).
- **Sense of Purpose**: Working towards common goals gives individuals a sense of purpose and direction (Hackman, 2002).
- **Support**: Groups offer emotional and practical support, helping members cope with stress and challenges (Cohen & Wills, 1985).
- **Sense of Belonging**: Being part of a group fosters a sense of belonging and identity, which is crucial for psychological well-being (Tajfel & Turner, 1986).
- **Assistance with Problems**: Groups provide a network of resources and assistance, enabling members to solve problems more effectively (Wheelan, 2009).

Team Requirements for Success

1. Clear Objectives and Terms

For a team to be successful, it must have clear objectives and terms. This clarity helps team members understand what they are supposed to achieve, the scope of their work, and how their efforts fit with other teams. According to Hackman (2002), clear goals are essential for team effectiveness as they provide direction and a basis for evaluating performance (Hackman, 2002).

2. Support from Management and Adequate Resources

Teams require support from management and adequate resources to function effectively. Without these, teams may struggle to achieve their goals. Management support includes providing necessary resources, removing obstacles, and offering guidance. Research by Kozlowski and Ilgen (2006) highlights that organizational support is crucial for team success, as it ensures that teams have the tools and environment needed to perform their tasks (Kozlowski & Ilgen, 2006).

3. A Base and Territory

Having a base or territory, such as a home ground for sports teams, can enhance team performance. This concept extends to virtual teams, which need a digital space where they can collaborate effectively. The sense of having a "home" can boost team morale and cohesion. Edmondson and Nembhard (2009) discuss how physical and virtual spaces can impact team dynamics and performance (Edmondson & Nembhard, 2009).

4. A Means of Identification

A team needs a name or other means of identification to be recognized as a distinct entity. This identification fosters a sense of belonging and pride among team members. The significance of a team name is supported by social identity theory, which suggests that identification with a group enhances cohesion and motivation (Tajfel & Turner, 1986).

5. Stability

Stability is crucial for maintaining team continuity and morale. Frequent changes in team composition can disrupt team dynamics and reduce effectiveness. Wheelan (2009) emphasizes that stable teams are more likely to develop strong cohesion and trust, which are essential for high performance (Wheelan, 2009).

6. Leadership

Effective leadership provides a focal point or "pivot" for a team. Leaders play a critical role in guiding the team, resolving conflicts, and maintaining motivation. Transformational leadership, which involves inspiring and motivating team members, is particularly effective in enhancing team performance (Hackman & Wageman, 2005).

Responsibilities of Team Members

Communication

Effective communication is a cornerstone of successful teamwork. Team members must communicate openly and frequently with both the team leader and other members. This ensures that everyone is aligned with the team's goals and aware of their roles and responsibilities. According to Salas, Sims, and Burke (2005), communication is critical for coordinating actions, sharing information, and building mutual understanding within teams (Salas, Sims, & Burke, 2005).

Sharing Work and Supporting Others

Team members are expected to share in the workload and support each other. This collaborative effort helps distribute tasks evenly and ensures that no single member is overwhelmed. Research by Kozlowski and Ilgen (2006) highlights the importance of mutual support in teams, noting that it enhances team cohesion and performance (Kozlowski & Ilgen, 2006).

Cooperation

Cooperation involves working harmoniously with other team members to achieve common goals. It requires a willingness to collaborate, share resources, and assist others when needed. Cooperative behavior is essential for maintaining a positive team environment and achieving collective success. Johnson and Johnson (2009) emphasize that cooperative teams are more effective and experience higher levels of satisfaction and productivity (Johnson & Johnson, 2009).

Contribution

Each team member should contribute their skills and knowledge to help achieve the team's objectives. This involves taking initiative, being proactive, and leveraging one's strengths for the benefit of the team. Hackman (2002) notes that individual contributions are vital for team success, as they bring diverse perspectives and expertise to the table (Hackman, 2002).

Team Development Stages

Bruce Tuckman's model of team development outlines five stages that teams typically go through: Forming, Storming, Norming, Performing, and Adjourning. Each stage has distinct characteristics and challenges.

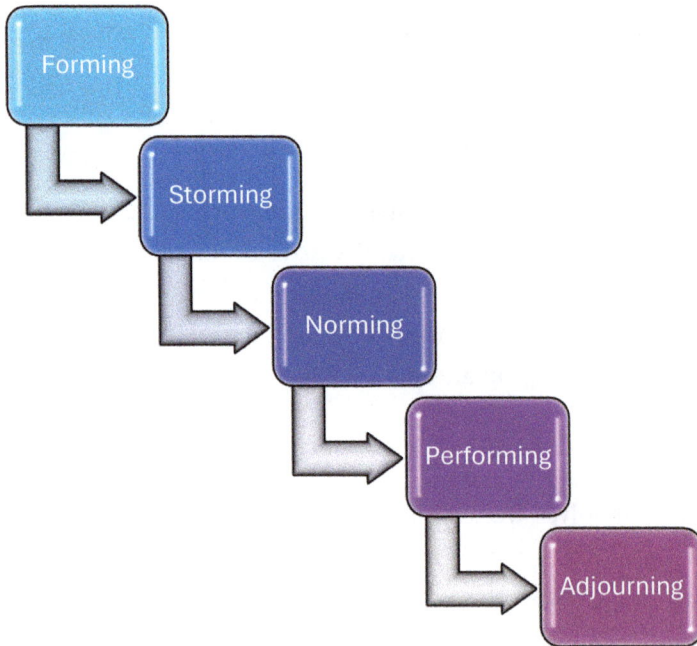

Figure 11.1: Team development stages

Forming

The Forming stage is the initial phase where team members come together and start to understand the team's purpose and structure. During this stage, members are often polite and positive, but also anxious about their roles and how they fit into the team. The primary focus is on orientation and getting acquainted. Members ask questions about the team's goals, their roles, and the expectations from them (Tuckman, 1965).

Storming

The Storming stage is marked by conflict and competition as individual personalities emerge. Team members may challenge the team's goals, leadership, and approaches. This stage is critical as it involves addressing conflicts and differences. If not managed well, teams can get stuck in this stage. Effective conflict resolution and the establishment of clear norms and roles are essential to move past this stage (Tuckman, 1965).

Norming

In the Norming stage, team members start to resolve their differences, appreciate colleagues' strengths, and respect the leader's authority. There is a sense of cohesion and unity as members agree on the team norms and expectations. Communication becomes more open and constructive, and the team starts to work more effectively towards its goals. This stage is characterized by increased cooperation and collaboration (Tuckman, 1965).

Performing

The Performing stage is where the team reaches optimal functionality. Members are confident, motivated, and able to handle decision-making without supervision. The team is highly productive, and roles are flexible as members take on various responsibilities as needed. This stage is marked by high levels of trust, autonomy, and efficiency in achieving the team's objectives (Tuckman, 1965).

Adjourning

The Adjourning stage, added later by Tuckman, involves the dissolution of the team after achieving its goals. This stage can be emotional as members reflect on their accomplishments and the end of their collaboration. It is important to acknowledge the team's efforts and provide closure. This stage may involve finalizing tasks, documenting outcomes, and celebrating the team's success (Tuckman & Jensen, 1977).

Factors Affecting Team Cohesiveness

Team Size

The size of a team can significantly impact its cohesiveness. Smaller teams tend to have higher levels of cohesion because members can interact more frequently and develop stronger interpersonal relationships. Larger teams, on the other hand, may struggle with coordination and communication, leading to lower cohesion (Wheelan, 2009).

Similarity of Work

Teams where members perform similar tasks often experience higher cohesion. This similarity fosters a shared understanding and mutual respect among team members. When team members have similar roles, they are more likely to empathize with each other's challenges and support one another (Kozlowski & Ilgen, 2006).

Background of Team Members

The background of team members, including their skills, experiences, and cultural backgrounds, can influence team cohesion. Diverse teams can benefit from a variety of perspectives and problem-solving approaches, but they may also face challenges in achieving cohesion if differences are not managed effectively (Bell et al., 2011).

Communication Ease

Effective communication is crucial for team cohesion. Teams that can communicate easily and frequently are more likely to develop strong bonds. Conversely, teams that face communication barriers, such as language differences or geographical dispersion, may experience feelings of isolation and separation, which can hinder cohesion (Gibson & Cohen, 2003).

Quality Team Members

Team Leader

The team leader plays a pivotal role in maintaining trust and support among team members, minimizing interpersonal conflict, leading meetings, directing activities towards goals, ensuring productive use of time, and representing the team to management (Hackman, 2002).

Team Facilitator

The team facilitator ensures equal participation, mediates and resolves conflicts, provides feedback and support to the team leader, and suggests problem-solving tools and techniques. This role is essential for maintaining a balanced and productive team environment (Salas, Sims, & Burke, 2005).

Team Member

Team members contribute by offering perspectives and ideas, actively participating in meetings, adhering to ground rules, completing assignments on time, and supporting the implementation of recommenda-tions. Their active engagement is crucial for the team's success (Johnson & Johnson, 2009).

Recorder

The recorder is responsible for taking minutes during meetings and distributing them to all team members. This role ensures that there is a clear and accurate record of discussions and decisions, which is vital for accountability and follow-up (Wheelan, 2009).

Timekeeper

The timekeeper helps manage the team's time during meetings, ensuring that discussions stay on track and that the team makes efficient use of its time. This role is important for maintaining productivity and focus (Hackman, 2002).

References

1. Baumeister, R. F., & Leary, M. R. (1995). The need to belong: Desire for interpersonal attachments as a fundamental human motivation. Psychological Bulletin, 117(3), 497-529. https://doi.org/10.1037/0033-2909.117.3.497

2. Bell, S. T., Villado, A. J., Lukasik, M. A., Belau, L., & Briggs, A. L. (2011). Getting specific about demographic diversity variable and team performance relationships: A meta-analysis. Journal of Management, 37(3), 709-743. https://doi.org/10.1177/0149206310365001

3. Bell, S. T., Villado, A. J., Lukasik, M. A., Belau, L., & Briggs, A. L. (2011). Getting specific about demographic diversity variable and team performance relationships: A meta-analysis. Journal of Management, 37(3), 709-743. https://doi.org/10.1177/0149206310365001

4. Cohen, S. G., & Bailey, D. E. (1997). What makes teams work: Group effectiveness research from the shop floor to the executive suite. Journal of Management, 23(3), 239-290. https://doi.org/10.1177/014920639702300303

5. Cohen, S., & Wills, T. A. (1985). Stress, social support, and the buffering hypothesis. Psychological Bulletin, 98(2), 310-357. https://doi.org/10.1037/0033-2909.98.2.310

6. Edmondson, A. C., & Nembhard, I. M. (2009). Product development and learning in project teams: The challenges are the benefits. Journal of Product Innovation Management, 26(2), 123-138. https://doi.org/10.1111/j.1540-5885.2009.00341.x

7. Gibson, C. B., & Cohen, S. G. (2003). Virtual teams that work: Creating conditions for virtual team effectiveness. Jossey-Bass.

8. Hackman, J. R. (2002). Leading teams: Setting the stage for great performances. Harvard Business School Press.

9. Hackman, J. R., & Wageman, R. (2005). A theory of team coaching. Academy of Management Review, 30(2), 269-287. https://doi.org/10.5465/amr.2005.16387885

10. Johnson, D. W., & Johnson, F. P. (2009). Joining together: Group theory and group skills (10th ed.). Pearson.

11. Kozlowski, S. W. J., & Ilgen, D. R. (2006). Enhancing the effectiveness of work groups and teams. Psychological Science in the Public Interest, 7(3), 77-124. https://doi.org/10.1111/j.1529-1006.2006.00030.x

12. Kozlowski, S. W. J., & Ilgen, D. R. (2006). Enhancing the effectiveness of work groups and teams. Psychological Science in the Public Interest, 7(3), 77-124. https://doi.org/10.1111/j.1529-1006.2006.00030.x

13. Mathieu, J. E., Maynard, M. T., Rapp, T., & Gilson, L. (2008). Team effectiveness 1997-2007: A review of recent advancements and a glimpse into the future. Journal of Management, 34(3), 410-476. https://doi.org/10.1177/0149206308316061

14. Morrison-Smith, S., & Ruiz, J. (2020). Challenges and barriers in virtual teams: A literature review. SN Applied Sciences, 2(1096). https://doi.org/10.1007/s42452-020-2801-5

15. National Academies of Sciences, Engineering, and Medicine. (2015). Enhancing the effectiveness of team science. The National Academies Press. https://doi.org/10.17226/19007

16. National Research Council. (2015). Enhancing the effectiveness of team science. The National Academies Press. https://doi.org/10.17226/19007

17. Salas, E., Sims, D. E., & Burke, C. S. (2005). Is there a "big five" in teamwork? Small Group Research, 36(5), 555-599. https://doi.org/10.1177/1046496405277134

18. Tajfel, H., & Turner, J. C. (1986). The social identity theory of intergroup behavior. In S. Worchel & W. G. Austin (Eds.), Psychology of intergroup relations (pp. 7-24). Nelson-Hall.

19. Tuckman, B. W. (1965). Developmental sequence in small groups. Psychological Bulletin, 63(6), 384-399. https://doi.org/10.1037/h0022100

20. Tuckman, B. W., & Jensen, M. A. C. (1977). Stages of small-group development revisited. Group & Organization Studies, 2(4), 419-427. https://doi.org/10.1177/105960117700200404

21. Wheelan, S. A. (2009). Creating effective teams: A guide for members and leaders. SAGE Publications.

Chapter 12

Regulatory and Compliance in Medical Quality.

What is Certification?

Certification in healthcare quality is a multifaceted process that applies to both individuals and facilities. It ensures that the certified entity, whether a person, unit, product, or facility, meets the established minimum standards required to perform specific activities or services (Agency for Healthcare Research and Quality, 2022). Certification can be seen as an "add-on" that enhances the credibility and capability of the certified entity.

People and Facilities

Both individuals and facilities can obtain certification. For individuals, certification often involves passing an exam that demonstrates their knowledge and skills in a specific area of healthcare. For example, a nurse might become certified in a specialty area such as oncology or pediatrics, which signifies that they have met the rigorous standards set by a certifying body (Centers for Medicare & Medicaid Services, 2021). Facilities, on the other hand, might be certified to perform certain types of procedures or to provide specific types of care, ensuring that they meet the necessary standards for quality and safety (Institute of Medicine, 2001).

Units and Products

Certification is not limited to people and facilities; it can also apply to units within a healthcare organization and to products used in healthcare. For instance, a laboratory unit within a hospital might be certified to conduct certain types of tests, ensuring that the tests are performed accurately and reliably (Rockit, 2022). Similarly, medical products such as surgical instruments or diagnostic devices can be certified to ensure they meet safety and efficacy standards.

Minimum Standards

The certification process involves assessing whether the entity meets the minimum standards required for certification. These standards are typically set by professional organizations or regulatory bodies and are designed to ensure that certified entities can provide high-quality, safe, and effective care (Agency for Healthcare Research and Quality, 2022). Meeting these standards often involves rigorous training, testing, and ongoing education.

Specific Activities or Services

Entities are certified to perform specific activities or services. This means that certification is not a one-size-fits-all process but is tailored to the specific functions that the entity will perform. For example, a healthcare facility might be certified to perform cardiac surgeries, indicating that it has the necessary equipment, trained personnel, and protocols in place to perform these surgeries safely and effectively (Centers for Medicare & Medicaid Services, 2021).

Add-On Qualification

Certification is often considered an add-on qualification. For individuals, it adds to their professional credentials, demonstrating their expertise in a particular area. For facilities and units, it adds to their reputation and credibility, showing that they meet high standards of quality and safety (Institute of Medicine, 2001). This additional qualification can be crucial in a competitive healthcare environment where patients and stakeholders are increasingly looking for assurances of quality.

What is Licensure?

Licensure in the context of healthcare quality and patient safety is a critical regulatory process. It involves assessing whether a facility, organization, or professional has met the minimum requirements necessary to engage in specific activities or provide certain services. This process ensures that only those who have demonstrated the requisite knowledge, skills, and competencies are allowed to operate within the healthcare system (World Health Organization, 2023).

To a Person or a Facility?

Licensure applies to both individuals and facilities. For individuals, such as doctors, nurses, and other healthcare professionals, licensure typically involves passing a standardized examination and meeting educational and training requirements. This process ensures that healthcare professionals are qualified to provide safe and effective care (Agency for Healthcare Research and Quality, 2024). For facilities, licensure involves meeting standards related to infrastructure, equipment, staffing, and operational procedures. This ensures that healthcare facilities can provide a safe environment for patient care (Centers for Medicare & Medicaid Services, 2021).

Both individuals and facilities must obtain licensure to operate legally within the healthcare system. This dual requirement helps maintain high standards of care and ensures that both the providers and the environments in which they work are equipped to deliver safe and effective healthcare services (Institute of Medicine, 2001).

The Process of Assessing Minimum Requirements

The licensure process involves a thorough assessment to determine whether the entity meets the established minimum requirements. These requirements are typically set by government entities or professional regulatory bodies and are designed to ensure a baseline level of quality and safety in healthcare delivery (World Health Organization, 2023). The assessment process may include inspections, audits, and reviews of documentation and performance data.

Engagement in Certain Activities

Once licensed, the entity—whether a person or a facility—is authorized to engage in specific activities or provide certain services. For example, a licensed physician can practice medicine, while a licensed hospital can offer inpatient and outpatient services. This authorization is crucial for ensuring that only qualified entities are involved in patient care (Agency for Healthcare Research and Quality, 2024).

Prohibition Without Licensure

Without licensure, individuals and facilities are prohibited from working or providing services or products within the healthcare system. This prohibition is essential for protecting patients from unqualified providers and unsafe facilities. It also helps maintain public trust in the healthcare system by ensuring that all providers meet established standards of quality and safety (Centers for Medicare & Medicaid Services, 2021).

Government Entity

Licensure is most often overseen by government entities, such as state health departments or national regulatory agencies. These entities are responsible for setting the standards, conducting assessments, and issuing licenses. They also have the authority to revoke or suspend licenses if the entity fails to maintain the required standards (Institute of Medicine, 2001).

Credentialing and Privileging

Credentialing and privileging are essential processes in healthcare quality and patient safety. They ensure that healthcare practitioners are qualified and competent to provide patient care services.

Who Will Be Included in This Process?

The credentialing and privileging process includes a wide range of healthcare professionals, not just surgeons. This process applies to physicians, dentists, visiting doctors, and new employees within a healthcare organization (Centers for Medicare & Medicaid Services, 2021). It ensures that all practitioners meet the necessary standards to provide safe and effective care.

Is It Only for Surgeons?

No, credentialing and privileging are not limited to surgeons. These processes apply to all healthcare practitioners, including primary care physicians, specialists, and allied health professionals. The goal is to ensure that all providers, regardless of their specialty, have the appropriate qualifications and competencies (Agency for Healthcare Research and Quality, 2024).

What About Dentists?

Dentists are also included in the credentialing and privileging process. They must undergo similar evaluations to verify their qualifications, licensure, education, training, and experience. This ensures that they are competent to perform dental procedures and provide patient care (World Health Organization, 2023).

What About Visiting Doctors?

Visiting doctors, or locum tenens, must also go through the credentialing and privileging process before they can provide care in a healthcare facility. This ensures that they meet the same standards as permanent staff and are qualified to deliver safe and effective care (Centers for Medicare & Medicaid Services, 2021).

Who Approves Them?

The approval of healthcare practitioners through credentialing and privileging is typically overseen by a credentialing committee within the healthcare organization. This committee reviews the practitioner's qualifications, verifies their credentials, and assesses their competence. The final approval is often granted by the organization's governing body or medical staff leadership (Agency for Healthcare Research and Quality, 2024).

What About New Employees?

New employees, including newly hired healthcare practitioners, must also undergo the credentialing and privileging process. This ensures that they meet the organization's standards for providing patient care and are qualified to perform their designated roles (World Health Organization, 2023).

Credentialing

Credentialing involves the evaluation of a clinician to become a member of the medical staff at an organization. This process includes obtaining, verifying, and assessing the qualifications of a healthcare practitioner. It determines if an individual can provide patient care services in or for a healthcare organization or network. Credentialing requires evidence of competence, current and relevant licensure, education, training, and experience. Additional criteria may be added by the healthcare organization to ensure comprehensive evaluation (Centers for Medicare & Medicaid Services, 2021).

Privileging

Privileging is the process by which a clinician is granted certain privileges based on their credentials. This includes determining the scope of procedures they are allowed to perform, such as invasive versus non-invasive procedures. Privileging ensures that the medical staff is qualified and permitted to perform specific clinical services within the organization, considering the availability of required resources (Agency for Healthcare Research and Quality, 2024).

What is Accreditation?

Accreditation is the process of assessing the quality of an organization to provide comparative information to the customer. It involves an objective evaluation by an independent body to ensure that the organization meets established standards of quality and safety (The Joint Commission, 2023). This process helps healthcare organizations measure, assess, and improve their performance to provide safe, high-quality care for their patients.

Accreditation of What?

Accreditation can apply to various entities within the healthcare system, including facilities, organizations, educational entities, and specific units, departments, or products.

Facilities

Healthcare facilities, such as hospitals, clinics, and long-term care facilities, can be accredited. This accreditation ensures that the facility meets the necessary standards for providing safe and effective patient care. The Joint Commission, for example, conducts on-site surveys to evaluate compliance with their standards, which cover important processes and organizational functions essential for high-quality care (The Joint Commission, 2023).

Organizations

Healthcare organizations, including health systems and networks, can also be accredited. This type of accreditation assesses the overall performance of the organization, including its governance, management, and operational processes. Accreditation helps organizations identify risks to quality and patient safety and encourages continuous improvement (The Joint Commission, 2023).

Educational Entities

Educational entities, such as medical schools and training programs, can be accredited to ensure they provide high-quality education and training to future healthcare professionals. Accreditation of educational programs ensures that graduates are competent to practice safely and effectively and are prepared for lifelong learning and further training (World Health Organization, 2023).

Units, Departments, or Products

Specific units or departments within a healthcare facility, such as a laboratory or radiology department, can be accredited. This ensures that these units meet the standards for performing specific functions and providing certain services. Additionally, medical products, such as surgical instruments or diagnostic devices, can be accredited to ensure they meet safety and efficacy standards (The Joint Commission, 2023).

Evolution of Healthcare Accreditation

1917: American College of Surgeons

The evolution of healthcare accreditation began in 1917 with the American College of Surgeons (ACS). The ACS initiated the Hospital Standardization Program, which was the first effort to improve the quality of care in hospitals by establishing minimum standards (The Joint Commission, 2023).

Hospital Standardization Program

The Hospital Standardization Program aimed to ensure that hospitals provided safe and effective care. This program laid the groundwork for modern accreditation processes by emphasizing the importance of standardized practices and continuous improvement in healthcare (The Joint Commission, 2023).

1952: Joint Commission (JCAH)

In 1952, the Joint Commission on Accreditation of Hospitals (JCAH) was established. This organization, now known as The Joint Commission, expanded the scope of accreditation to include a broader range of healthcare facilities and services. The JCAH set rigorous standards for healthcare organizations and conducted regular evaluations to ensure compliance (The Joint Commission, 2023).

1958-1990: Few Countries with Accreditation

Between 1958 and 1990, only a few countries had established accreditation programs. During this period, accreditation was primarily a North American phenomenon, with limited adoption in other regions. However, the foundational principles and benefits of accreditation began to gain recognition globally (IQAS, 2023).

1990-Present: 50+ Countries

Since the 1990s, the number of countries with healthcare accreditation programs has grown significantly. Today, over 50 countries have implemented accreditation systems to improve the quality and safety of healthcare services. This global expansion reflects the increasing recognition of accreditation as a valuable tool for enhancing healthcare quality (IQAS, 2023).

Next Generation of Accreditation

The next generation of accreditation is expected to be shaped by ongoing technological advancements, globalization, and a continued emphasis on outcomes. Innovations such as artificial intelligence and machine learning are anticipated to enhance the accreditation process by providing more nuanced insights into quality and performance (IQAS, 2023).

Accrediting Organizations

United States

The Joint Commission (TJC)

The Joint Commission (TJC) accredits a variety of healthcare organizations (HCOs) including hospitals, ambulatory care centers, behavioral health care, home care, and laboratory services. TJC's accreditation process involves evaluating healthcare organizations against rigorous performance standards to ensure quality and safety in patient care (The Joint Commission, n.d.).

National Committee for Quality Assurance (NCQA)

The National Committee for Quality Assurance (NCQA) focuses on improving healthcare quality through the administration of evidence-based standards, measures, programs, and accreditation. NCQA accredits health plans, managed behavioral healthcare organizations, and other healthcare entities. Their programs include the Healthcare Effectiveness Data and Information Set (HEDIS) and the Patient-Centered Medical Home (PCMH) recognition (NCQA, n.d.).

Accreditation Association for Ambulatory Health Care (AAAHC)

The Accreditation Association for Ambulatory Health Care (AAAHC) specializes in accrediting ambulatory healthcare organizations. This includes ambulatory surgery centers, office-based surgery centers, primary care practices, and student health centers. AAAHC's accreditation emphasizes continuous improvement and adherence to nationally recognized standards (AAAHC, n.d.).

URAC

URAC, originally known as the Utilization Review Accreditation Commission, accredits a wide range of healthcare organizations, including health plans, pharmacies, telehealth providers, and ambulatory care centers. URAC's accreditation programs are designed to promote healthcare quality through leadership, accreditation, measurement, and innovation (URAC, n.d.).

Commission on Accreditation of Rehabilitation Facilities (CARF)

The Commission on Accreditation of Rehabilitation Facilities (CARF) accredits rehabilitation facilities and other health and human services providers. CARF's accreditation process involves a consultative peer review and is designed to improve the quality of services and enhance the lives of the persons served (CARF International, n.d.).

International Accrediting Organizations

Det Norske Veritas (DNV)

Det Norske Veritas (DNV) introduced the National Integrated Accreditation for Healthcare Organizations (NIAHO) in 2008. DNV's accreditation integrates ISO 9001 quality management standards with the Medicare Conditions of Participation, providing a comprehensive approach to hospital accreditation (DNV, n.d.).

Healthcare Facilities Accreditation Program (HFAP)

The Healthcare Facilities Accreditation Program (HFAP) is one of the oldest accrediting organizations in the United States, originally part of the American Osteopathic Association. HFAP accredits hospitals, ambulatory surgery centers, clinical laboratories, and other healthcare facilities, focusing on patient safety and quality of care (ACHC International, n.d.).

Accreditation Canada

Accreditation Canada provides accreditation services to healthcare organizations in Canada and internationally. Their Qmentum program is designed to help organizations meet national and international standards, improve quality, and ensure patient safety. Accreditation Canada works with Health Standards Organization (HSO) to develop and maintain their standards (Accreditation Canada, n.d.).

Australian Council on Healthcare Standards (ACHS)

The Australian Council on Healthcare Standards (ACHS) is an independent, not-for-profit organization dedicated to improving the quality of healthcare in Australia. ACHS provides accreditation services to a wide range of healthcare organizations, including hospitals and primary care providers, through programs such as the National Safety and Quality Health Service (NSQHS) Standards (ACHS, n.d.).

Saudi Central Board for Accreditation of Healthcare Institutions (CBAHI)

The Saudi Central Board for Accreditation of Healthcare Institutions (CBAHI) is the official agency responsible for accrediting healthcare facilities in Saudi Arabia. CBAHI's accreditation programs are designed to improve the quality of healthcare services and ensure compliance with national and international standards (CBAHI, n.d.).

ACQH Kazakhstan

ACQH Kazakhstan is involved in accrediting healthcare organizations in Central Asian countries and not limited to Kazakhstan, Russia, Uzbekistan , and Kyrgyzstan. It focuses on improving healthcare quality and patient safety through adherence to established standards and continuous improvement processes.

Other Nations

Several other nations, including France, Japan, and South Africa, have their own accrediting bodies that ensure healthcare organizations meet specific quality and safety standards. These organizations work to improve healthcare delivery and patient outcomes within their respective countries.

Scope of Accreditation

Hospital

Hospital accreditation is a comprehensive evaluation process that ensures hospitals meet specific standards of quality and safety. Accredited hospitals are recognized for their commitment to providing high-quality patient care and maintaining a safe environment. The Joint Commission (TJC) is one of the primary accrediting bodies for hospitals in the United States, offering accreditation that covers a wide range of services, including inpatient care, surgical services, and emergency care (The Joint Commission, n.d.).

Ambulatory Care Facilities

Ambulatory care facilities provide medical services on an outpatient basis, without the need for hospital admission. These facilities include primary health care (PHC) centers, clinics, medical groups, and specialized centers such as surgi-centers and emergency rooms (ER).

- **PHC Centers**: Primary health care centers offer a broad range of services, including preventive care, diagnosis, and treatment of common illnesses. They are often the first point of contact for patients seeking medical attention (The Joint Commission, n.d.).
- **Clinics**: Clinics provide specialized medical services, often focusing on specific areas such as dermatology, cardiology, or orthopedics. They offer both diagnostic and therapeutic services (The Joint Commission, n.d.).
- **Medical Groups**: Medical groups consist of multiple healthcare providers who work together to offer comprehensive care. These groups can include general practitioners, specialists, and other healthcare professionals (The Joint Commission, n.d.).
- **Surgi-Centers and ER Centers**: Surgical centers (surgi-centers) and emergency rooms (ER centers) provide specialized surgical and emergency care services. These facilities are equipped to handle a variety of medical emergencies and surgical procedures (The Joint Commission, n.d.).

Clinical Labs

Clinical laboratories play a crucial role in the diagnosis and treatment of diseases. They perform a wide range of tests on clinical specimens to obtain information about the health of a patient. Accreditation for clinical labs ensures that they meet high standards of quality and accuracy in their testing processes. The International Laboratory Accreditation Cooperation (ILAC) provides guidelines for the formulation of scopes of accreditation for laboratories, ensuring they adhere to international standards (ILAC, 2010).

Health Maintenance Organizations (HMOs)

Health Maintenance Organizations (HMOs) provide managed care for health insurance policyholders. They offer a range of healthcare services through a network of providers. Accreditation for HMOs focuses on ensuring that these organizations provide high-quality care, maintain adequate provider networks, and meet regulatory requirements. The National Committee for Quality Assurance (NCQA) is a key accrediting body for HMOs, providing standards and guidelines to improve healthcare quality (NCQA, n.d.).

Rehabilitation Facilities

Rehabilitation facilities offer specialized care for individuals recovering from injuries, surgeries, or illnesses. These facilities provide physical, occupational, and speech therapy to help patients regain their functional abilities. The Commission on Accreditation of Rehabilitation Facilities (CARF) accredits rehabilitation facilities, ensuring they meet rigorous standards for quality and patient safety (CARF International, n.d.).

Psychiatric Care Facilities

Psychiatric care facilities provide treatment for individuals with mental health disorders. These facilities offer a range of services, including inpatient and outpatient care, counseling, and medication management. Accreditation for psychiatric care facilities ensures that they provide safe and effective treatment. The Joint Commission accredits psychiatric hospitals and other behavioral health care organizations, focusing on standards that promote patient safety and quality of care (The Joint Commission, n.d.).

Funding of Healthcare Accreditation

Government/MOH

Government funding, often through Ministries of Health (MOH), is a significant source of support for healthcare accreditation programs. For example, the Centers for Disease Control and Prevention (CDC) provides funding to the Public Health Accreditation Board (PHAB) to support the accreditation of public health departments in the United States (CDC, n.d.). This funding helps ensure that health departments meet national standards and improve their performance.

Grants

Grants from various organizations, including federal agencies and private foundations, are crucial for funding healthcare accreditation. The CDC, for instance, offers grants to support the operations and continuous improvement of national voluntary accreditation programs for state, tribal, local, and territorial health departments (CDC, n.d.). These grants help cover the costs associated with maintaining and enhancing accreditation standards.

Survey Fees

Survey fees are charged by accrediting bodies to cover the costs of the accreditation process. These fees typically include expenses for on-site evaluations, travel, and administrative costs. The Joint Commission, for example, charges an on-site survey fee that varies based on the size and type of the organization being accredited (The Joint Commission, n.d.). These fees are essential for funding the comprehensive evaluation process that ensures healthcare organizations meet established standards.

Membership Fees

Membership fees are another common source of funding for accrediting organizations. Institutions seeking accreditation often pay annual membership dues, which support the accrediting body's operations and services. For instance, the Public Health Accreditation Board (PHAB) charges fees based on the size of the jurisdictional population served by the health department (PHAB, n.d.). These fees help sustain the accreditation process and provide resources for continuous improvement.

Publications/Training/Education

Accrediting organizations generate revenue through the sale of publications, training programs, and educational services. These resources are designed to help institutions understand and meet accreditation standards. The CDC, for example, provides various publications and training materials to support health departments in their accreditation efforts (CDC, n.d.). These activities not only generate income but also enhance the quality and effectiveness of the accreditation process.

Board Member Organization Support

Support from board member organizations is another vital funding source. Board members often represent institutions or organizations that contribute financially to the accrediting body. This support can come in the form of direct financial contributions or in-kind services. For example, the Public Health Accreditation Board (PHAB) receives support from various public health organizations that are represented on its board (CDC, n.d.). This support helps ensure the sustainability and effectiveness of the accreditation program.

Consulting

Consulting services provided by accrediting organizations can also be a significant source of funding. These services include offering expert advice and assistance to institutions seeking accreditation. For instance, consulting firms like BerryDunn provide public health consulting services to help health departments prepare for accreditation, manage grants, and improve their operations (BerryDunn, n.d.). These consulting services not only generate revenue but also help institutions achieve and sustain high standards of quality.

Purpose of Healthcare Accreditation

Demand of the Customer

Healthcare accreditation is often driven by the demand of customers who seek assurance of quality and safety in healthcare services. Customers, including patients and their families, expect healthcare organizations to meet high standards of care. Accreditation provides external validation that these standards are being met, thereby building trust and confidence among stakeholders (Accreditation Council, n.d.).

A Forum for Measuring Performance

Accreditation serves as a forum for measuring the performance of healthcare organizations. It involves the use of standardized performance measures to evaluate the quality of care provided. For example, The Joint Commission (TJC) has developed core performance measures that hospitals must meet to achieve accreditation. These measures help organizations assess their performance and identify areas for improvement (The Joint Commission, n.d.).

Standardization and Variance Control

Standardization and variance control are key purposes of accreditation. By adhering to established standards, healthcare organizations can reduce variability in care delivery, ensuring consistent and high-quality services. This process involves implementing best practices and protocols that are recognized and validated by accrediting bodies (Hussein et al., 2021).

Benchmarking

Benchmarking is a critical component of accreditation, allowing healthcare organizations to compare their performance against industry standards and best practices. This process helps identify areas where improvements are needed and promotes the adoption of effective strategies used by top-performing organizations (Willmington et al., 2022).

Report Cards

Accreditation often involves the use of report cards, which provide a summary of an organization's performance on various quality measures. These report cards are made available to the public, helping consumers make informed decisions about their healthcare providers. For instance, the National Committee for Quality Assurance (NCQA) publishes report cards for health plans, highlighting their performance on key quality indicators (RAND, 2002).

Quality Improvement

One of the primary purposes of accreditation is to drive continuous quality improvement. Accrediting bodies like The Joint Commission use the accreditation process to identify areas for improvement and provide guidance on best practices. This ongoing focus on quality helps healthcare organizations enhance their services and patient outcomes (The Joint Commission, n.d.).

Positive Competition

Accreditation fosters positive competition among healthcare organizations. By striving to meet accreditation standards, organizations are motivated to improve their performance and achieve recognition for their efforts. This competitive environment encourages innovation and excellence in healthcare delivery (PowerDMS, 2020).

Reward and Recognition

Accreditation provides a framework for rewarding and recognizing healthcare organizations that meet high standards of care. Achieving accreditation is a mark of excellence that can enhance an organization's reputation and attract patients. It also serves as a motivational tool for staff, who take pride in working for an accredited institution (Life QI, 2021).

To Meet the Needs and Expectation of the Customer

Meeting the needs and expectations of customers is a fundamental purpose of accreditation. Healthcare organizations seek accreditation to demonstrate their commitment to providing high-quality care that meets the expectations of patients and their families. This focus on customer satisfaction is central to the accreditation process (The Joint Commission, n.d.).

Efficiency

Accreditation helps healthcare organizations improve their efficiency by streamlining processes and reducing waste. Accredited organizations often implement standardized protocols and best practices that enhance operational efficiency and reduce costs. This focus on efficiency ultimately benefits patients by improving the quality and timeliness of care (Jha, 2018).

Effectiveness

The effectiveness of healthcare services is a key focus of accreditation. Accrediting bodies evaluate the outcomes of care provided by healthcare organizations to ensure they are achieving the desired results. This emphasis on effectiveness helps organizations continuously improve their services and achieve better patient outcomes (The Joint Commission, n.d.).

References:

1. Accreditation Canada. (n.d.). https://www.accreditation.ca
2. Accreditation Commission for Health Care International (ACHC International). (n.d.). https://www.achcinternational.org/hfap/
3. Accreditation Council. (n.d.). The purpose of accreditation. https://accreditationcouncil.org/Programs/The-Purpose-of-Accreditation
4. Agency for Healthcare Research and Quality. (2022). Six domains of healthcare quality. https://www.ahrq.gov/talkingquality/measures/six-domains.html
5. Agency for Healthcare Research and Quality. (2024). Ensuring patient and workforce safety culture in healthcare. https://psnet.ahrq.gov/perspective/ensuring-patient-and-workforce-safety-culture-healthcare
6. Australian Council on Healthcare Standards (ACHS). (n.d.). https://www.achs. org.au
7. BerryDunn. (n.d.). Public Health Consulting. https://www.berrydunn.com/industries/public-health
8. CARF International. (n.d.). https://www.carf.org
9. CBAHI. (n.d.). https://portal.cbahi.gov.sa/english/home
10. Centers for Disease Control and Prevention (CDC). (n.d.). National Accreditation Program Support Funding. https://www.cdc.gov/public-health-gateway/php/funding/accreditation-support.html
11. Centers for Medicare & Medicaid Services. (2021). Quality measures: How they are developed, used, & maintained. https://www.cms.gov/sites/default/files/2021-09/Quality-Measures-How-They-Are-Developed-Used-Maintained.pdf
12. Det Norske Veritas (DNV). (n.d.). https://www.dnv.com/services/hospital-accreditation-7516/
13. Hussein, M., Pavlova, M., Ghalwash, M., & Groot, W. (2021). The impact of hospital accreditation on the quality of healthcare: A systematic literature review. BMC Health Services Research, 21(1057). https://bmchealthservres.biomedcentral.com/articles/10.1186/s12913-021-07097-6
14. Institute of Medicine. (2001). Crossing the quality chasm: A new health system for the 21st century. Washington, D.C: National Academy Press.
15. International Laboratory Accreditation Cooperation (ILAC). (2010). Guideline for the Formulation of Scopes of Accreditation for Laboratories.

https://european-accreditation.org/wp-content/uploads/2018/10/ILAC_G18_04_2010.pdf

16. IQAS. (2023). The evolution of accreditation – A journey towards quality assurance. https://www.iqascorp.com/post/the-evolution-of-accreditation-a-journey-towards-quality-assurance

17. Jha, A. K. (2018). Accreditation, quality, and making hospital care better. JAMA, 320(23), 2410-2411. doi:10.1001/jama.2018.18810

18. Life QI. (2021). Reward and recognition as motivators in healthcare. https://blog.lifeqisystem.com/rewards-recognition-as-motivation-healthcare

19. National Committee for Quality Assurance (NCQA). (n.d.). https://www.ncqa.org

20. PowerDMS. (2020). Impact of accreditation on quality in healthcare. https://www.powerdms.com/policy-learning-center/impact-of-accreditation-on-quality-in-healthcare

21. Public Health Accreditation Board (PHAB). (n.d.). Fees. https://phaboard.org/accreditation-recognition/fees/

22. RAND. (2002). Report cards for health care: Is anyone checking them? https://www.rand.org/pubs/research_briefs/RB4544.html

23. Rockit. (2022). Data quality in healthcare: A comprehensive guide to improving. https://rockitteam.com/blogs/data-quality-in-healthcare-guide/

24. The Joint Commission. (2023). History of The Joint Commission. https://www.jointcommission.org/who-we-are/facts-about-the-joint-commission/history-of-the-joint-commission/

25. The Joint Commission. (n.d.). https://www.jointcommission.org

26. The Joint Commission. (n.d.). Accreditation process overview fact sheet. https://www.jointcommission.org/resources/news-and-multimedia/fact-sheets/facts-about-accreditation-process-overview/

27. The Joint Commission. (n.d.). Hospital Accreditation Pricing. https://www.jointcommission.org/what-we-offer/accreditation/health-care-settings/hospital/learn/pricing/

28. URAC. (n.d.). https://www.urac.org

29. Willmington, C., Belardi, P., Murante, A. M., & Vainieri, M. (2022). The contribution of benchmarking to quality improvement in healthcare: A systematic literature review. BMC Health Services Research, 22(139). https://bmchealthservres.biomedcentral. com/articles/10.1186/s12913-022-07467-8

30. World Health Organization. (2023). Patient safety.
https://www.who.int/news-room/fact-sheets/detail/patient-safety

Chapter 13

Health Information Management

Definition of Health Information Systems:

Health Information Systems (HIS) is a multidisciplinary field that leverages information technology to enhance healthcare services, quality, efficiency, and effectiveness. HIS encompasses various components, including electronic health records (EHRs), health information exchanges (HIEs), and other technologies that facilitate the management and exchange of health information (Wager, Lee, & Glaser, 2017).

The primary goal of HIS is to improve patient care by ensuring that accurate and up-to-date information is available to healthcare providers. This includes the use of EHRs, which allow for the digital recording of patient information, making it easier to access and share across different healthcare settings (McGonigle & Mastrian, 2021). Additionally, HIS supports clinical decision-making by providing tools and data that help healthcare professionals make informed decisions (Hebda & Czar, 2013).

HIS also plays a crucial role in public health by enabling the collection and analysis of health data on a large scale. This data can be used to monitor disease outbreaks, track health trends, and inform public health policies (Yasnoff et al., 2001). Furthermore, HIS contributes to the efficiency of healthcare operations by streamlining administrative processes, reducing paperwork, and minimizing errors (Tan & Payton, 2010).

In summary, HIS is a vital component of modern healthcare, integrating technology to improve the delivery and management of health services, ultimately enhancing patient outcomes and operational efficiency.

Distinction between data and information:

In healthcare, the distinction between data and information is crucial for effective decision-making and patient care. The progression from data to wisdom involves several stages: data, information, knowledge, and wisdom.

Data are the raw, unprocessed facts and figures that are collected and stored in a structured format. These can include numbers, symbols, measurements, and statistics. For example, a patient's temperature reading or blood pressure measurement is considered data (American Institute for Healthcare Management, 2024).

Information is derived from data when it is processed, organized, or structured in a way that makes it meaningful and useful. In healthcare, this could involve interpreting a series of temperature readings to determine if a patient has a fever. Information is essential for making informed decisions and providing effective care (Healthcare IT Today, 2019).

Knowledge is created when information is combined with experience and context to form a deeper understanding. For instance, a healthcare provider uses information about a patient's symptoms and medical history to diagnose an illness. Knowledge allows healthcare professionals to apply information in practical, real-world scenarios (Healthcare IT Today, 2019).

Wisdom is the ability to make sound judgments and decisions based on knowledge. In healthcare, wisdom involves using knowledge to provide the best possible care for patients, considering both clinical evidence and individual patient needs. It represents the highest level of understanding and application (American Institute for Healthcare Management, 2024).

In summary, data are the foundational elements that, when processed into information, contribute to the development of knowledge and ultimately wisdom in healthcare settings. This progression is essential for effective decision-making and high-quality patient care.

Components of a Health Information System

Hardware

Hardware is the physical component of a Health Information System (HIS) and includes devices such as servers, workstations, and network devices. These components are essential for the storage, processing, and transmission of health data. Servers are used to store large amounts of data and run applications that manage health information. Workstations are used by healthcare professionals to access and input data. Network devices, such as routers and switches, ensure that data can be transmitted securely and efficiently across the healthcare network (Scopic, 2024).

Software

Software in a HIS includes the applications and programs that process and manage health information. This can range from electronic health records (EHR) systems to specialized software for medical imaging, laboratory information systems, and healthcare analytics platforms. Software is crucial for the automation of data processing, ensuring that health information is accurate, up-to-date, and accessible to authorized users. It also includes security software to protect sensitive health data from unauthorized access and breaches (Health IT Workforce Curriculum, 2012).

Customers

Customers of a HIS include a wide range of stakeholders such as healthcare providers, patients, and public health agencies. Healthcare providers use HIS to improve patient care by accessing comprehensive and accurate patient information. Patients benefit from HIS by having better access to their health records and being able to participate more actively in their care.

Public health agencies use HIS to monitor health trends, manage public health programs, and respond to health emergencies (KNBBS, 2023).

Difference between EHR and EMR

Electronic Health Record

An Electronic Health Record (EHR) is a systematized collection of patient and population health information stored electronically in a digital format. EHRs are designed to be shared across different healthcare settings, providing real-time, patient-centered records that make information available instantly whenever and wherever it is needed (HealthIT.gov, 2024). These records can include a patient's medical history, diagnoses, medications, immunization dates, allergies, radiology images, and laboratory test results (CMS, 2024). The primary goal of EHRs is to improve the quality of care by ensuring that health information is accurate, up-to-date, and accessible to authorized users.

Electronic Medical Record

An Electronic Medical Record (EMR) is a digital version of a patient's paper chart and is a subset of the EHR. EMRs contain the medical and treatment history of patients within a single practice and are primarily used by healthcare providers for diagnosis and treatment (USF Health Online, 2024). Unlike EHRs, which are designed to be shared across different healthcare settings, EMRs are typically used within one healthcare organization. EMRs include general information such as medical history, diagnoses, medications, allergies, lab results, and treatment plans (HealthIT.gov, 2024). They serve as a data source for EHRs, providing detailed and comprehensive patient information that can be integrated into the broader EHR system.

Barriers to Implementation of EHR/EMR

Data Security

Data security is a significant barrier to the implementation of Electronic Health Records (EHR) and Electronic Medical Records (EMR). Healthcare organizations must ensure that patient data is protected from unauthorized access and breaches. Cybersecurity threats and potential unauthorized access to EHR data cause apprehension about privacy protections (Calysta EMR, 2023). Safeguarding patient data is a top concern, and healthcare providers must implement robust security measures to protect sensitive health information (HealthIT.gov, 2024).

Data Entry Challenges

Data entry challenges are another barrier to the successful implementation of EHR/EMR systems. The process of entering data into EHR systems can be cumbersome and time-consuming for healthcare providers. A clinician's work process may make it hard or impossible to appropriately enter the desired EHR data, leading to errors and inefficiencies (American Medical Association, 2023). For example, a clinician might choose the wrong frequency for a drug to be administered due to changes in the order of options in the EHR system (American Medical Association, 2023).

Cost

The cost of implementing EHR/EMR systems is a major barrier for many healthcare organizations. The initial cost of adopting an EHR system can be substantial, including expenses for hardware, software, training, and ongoing maintenance (SelectHub, 2024). For instance, the average EHR implementation cost for a five-physician practice is estimated to be $162,000, with $85,000 in maintenance costs (SelectHub, 2024). These high costs can be prohibitive, especially for smaller practices.

Reliability

Reliability issues can also hinder the adoption of EHR/EMR systems. Healthcare providers need systems that are consistently available and perform reliably. Technical issues, such as system downtime and software bugs, can disrupt clinical workflows and negatively impact patient care (American Medical Association, 2023). Additionally, the lack of technical support once the EMR has launched can further exacerbate these reliability concerns (Boonstra & Broekhuis, 2010).

Productivity Impact

The implementation of EHR/EMR systems can have a significant impact on productivity. Healthcare providers often experience a decrease in productivity as they adapt to new systems and workflows. For example, physicians may spend more time entering data into the EHR, which can reduce the time available for patient care (National Center for Health Statistics, 2012). This productivity loss can be a major deterrent to the adoption of EHR/EMR systems.

Integration of Information Resources

Integrating EHR/EMR systems with other health information systems is a complex challenge. The lack of interoperability between different systems can hinder the seamless exchange of health information. Data standardization and the integration of diverse health IT systems, such as practice management systems and state registries, are essential for improving healthcare efficiency and patient outcomes (CAQH, 2023). However, achieving this integration requires significant effort and investment.

Integration of Information Resources

Integration of information resources in Electronic Health Records (EHR) and Electronic Medical Records (EMR) systems is crucial for enhancing healthcare delivery. This process involves connecting various digital systems and applications to enable seamless data sharing and communication. Effective integration ensures that healthcare providers have access to comprehensive patient information, which improves care coordination and decision-making (Langate, 2023). For instance, integrating EMR systems with laboratory information systems allows for the efficient management of lab data, enabling quick access to test results and better patient outcomes (SelectHub, 2024).

Management of Information

Confidentiality of Information Release of Information

Confidentiality is a fundamental aspect of managing health information. The release of patient information must be handled with utmost care to protect patient privacy. According to the Health Insurance Portability and Accountability Act (HIPAA), patient information should only be released with the patient's written consent or as permitted by law (HHS.gov, 2024). This ensures that sensitive health data is disclosed only to authorized individuals or organizations.

A written consent form is required for an organization to release patient information to anyone outside the organization. This form must include several key elements to ensure that the release of information is properly documented and authorized. These elements include:

- **Patient's name**: Clearly identifying the patient whose information is being released.
- **Name of individual/organization requesting information**: Specifying who is requesting the information.
- **Reason for release of information**: Explaining why the information is being requested.
- **Anticipated use of information released**: Describing how the information will be used.
- **Exact material to be released**: Detailing what specific information will be disclosed.
- **Time that the release of information is valid**: Indicating the period during which the release is valid.
- **Documentation that information is released only to the individual/organization above**: Ensuring that the information is only shared with the specified party.

- **Signature and date of the patient or legal representative**: Obtaining the patient's or their legal representative's signature and date to validate the consent (American Medical Association, 2012).

Who is authorized to receive patient information?

In the context of healthcare, the Health Insurance Portability and Accountability Act (HIPAA) outlines specific guidelines regarding who is authorized to receive and access patient information. The following entities and individuals are typically authorized:

Governing Body: The governing body of a healthcare organization, such as a hospital board, is responsible for overseeing the organization's operations and ensuring compliance with legal and regulatory requirements. This body has the authority to access patient information as necessary to fulfill its oversight responsibilities (U.S. Department of Health and Human Services [HHS], 2024).

Organization Director: The director or chief executive officer of a healthcare organization has the authority to access patient information to manage and direct the organization's operations effectively. This includes ensuring that patient care is delivered in accordance with established standards and regulations (HHS, 2024).

Healthcare Personnel Involved in the Care of the Patient: Healthcare providers directly involved in a patient's care, such as doctors, nurses, and allied health professionals, are authorized to access patient information. This access is necessary to provide appropriate and effective care (HHS, 2024).

Individuals Responsible for Quality Improvement Activities: Personnel involved in quality improvement activities within a healthcare organization are authorized to access patient information. This access is essential for monitoring and improving the quality of care provided to patients (HHS, 2024).

Individuals in the Medical Records Department: Staff members in the medical records department are responsible for maintaining and managing patient records. They are authorized to access patient information to ensure that records are accurate, complete, and available for authorized use (HHS, 2024).

General HIS Principles

IT is a Support Service: Information Technology (IT) in healthcare information systems (HIS) is fundamentally a support service. It provides the necessary infrastructure and tools to facilitate the efficient operation of healthcare services. IT supports clinical and administrative processes by ensuring that data is accessible, secure, and accurate (Smith & Jones, 2023).

IT Must Address Customer Needs: IT services in healthcare must be designed to meet the needs of their users, which include healthcare providers, patients, and administrative staff. This involves understanding the specific requirements of these stakeholders and developing solutions that enhance their ability to deliver and receive care. For instance, electronic health records (EHRs) must be user-friendly and tailored to the workflows of healthcare providers to improve patient care (Brown, 2022).

IT Cannot Drive the Business Process: While IT is crucial for the support and enhancement of healthcare services, it should not dictate the business processes. Instead, IT should be adaptable to the needs and strategies of the healthcare organization. The primary focus should be on improving patient outcomes and operational efficiency, rather than allowing technology to determine the direction of healthcare practices (Johnson, 2021).

Computers & HIS Functions

Quality Improvement and Risk Management: Computers in healthcare information systems (HIS) play a crucial role in quality improvement and risk management. They enable the collection, analysis, and reporting of data related to patient safety and care quality. This data-driven approach helps healthcare organizations identify areas for improvement and implement strategies to mitigate risks (Holmgren et al., 2023).

Decision Making: HIS supports clinical decision-making by providing healthcare professionals with access to comprehensive patient data and evidence-based guidelines. Decision support systems (DSS) integrated into HIS can offer real-time alerts and recommendations, enhancing the accuracy and efficiency of clinical decisions (Holmgren et al., 2023).

Patient Registration: Computers streamline the patient registration process by automating data entry and verification. This reduces errors, speeds up the registration process, and ensures that accurate patient information is available throughout the healthcare system (Smith & Jones, 2023).

Utilization Management: HIS facilitates utilization management by tracking the use of healthcare services and resources. This helps healthcare providers ensure that patients receive appropriate care while avoiding unnecessary tests and procedures, ultimately improving cost-efficiency (Brown, 2022).

Program Planning and Evaluation: Computers assist in program planning and evaluation by providing tools for data analysis and reporting. Healthcare organizations can use HIS to monitor program outcomes, assess effectiveness, and make data-driven decisions to enhance healthcare delivery (Johnson, 2021).

External Reporting: HIS enables healthcare organizations to comply with external reporting requirements by automating the collection and submission of data to regulatory bodies. This ensures that organizations meet legal and accreditation standards while maintaining transparency and accountability (Smith & Jones, 2023).

Research: Computers in HIS support healthcare research by providing access to large datasets and advanced analytical tools. Researchers can use HIS to conduct studies, analyze trends, and generate insights that contribute to medical knowledge and improve patient care (Brown, 2022).

Education: HIS enhances education and training for healthcare professionals by offering access to up-to-date information, clinical guidelines, and educational resources. This supports continuous learning and helps healthcare providers stay informed about the latest developments in their field (Johnson, 2021).

Clinical HIS Functions

Morbidity: Healthcare information systems (HIS) track morbidity rates by collecting and analyzing data on the incidence and prevalence of diseases within a population. This information helps healthcare providers identify trends, allocate resources, and develop targeted interventions to reduce disease burden (Mainz, 2003).

Mortality: HIS are essential for monitoring mortality rates, providing data on the number of deaths and their causes. This data is crucial for evaluating the effectiveness of healthcare interventions and identifying areas needing improvement. Accurate mortality data helps in formulating public health policies and improving patient outcomes (DesHarnais et al., 2023).

Complications: HIS track complications arising from medical treatments and procedures. By analyzing this data, healthcare organizations can identify patterns and implement strategies to minimize risks and improve patient safety. This function is vital for maintaining high standards of care and reducing adverse events (Holmgren et al., 2023).

Readmissions: HIS monitor hospital readmission rates, which are often used as indicators of healthcare quality. High readmission rates can signal issues with the initial care or discharge processes. HIS data helps healthcare providers develop interventions to reduce unnecessary readmissions, thereby improving patient care and reducing costs (Zook & Moore, 1980).

Clinical Indicators: Clinical indicators are specific measures used to assess the quality and performance of healthcare services. HIS collect and analyze data on various clinical indicators, such as infection rates, surgical outcomes, and patient satisfaction. This information is used to monitor performance, guide quality improvement initiatives, and ensure compliance with regulatory standards (Mainz, 2003).

Functions and Assistance of Health Information Systems (HIS) in Administrative Tasks

Accounts Payable

Accounts payable (AP) in healthcare involves managing the hospital's obligations to pay off short-term debts to its suppliers and creditors. This includes processing invoices, verifying transaction details, and ensuring timely payments to avoid late fees and maintain good supplier relationships. Effective AP management is crucial for maintaining the financial health of the institution and ensuring that all operational needs are met without interruption (Velvet Jobs, 2024). HIS can assist in automating these processes, reducing manual errors, and improving efficiency (Quadient, 2024).

Patient Accounting

Patient accounting refers to the financial services related to patient care, including billing, collections, and financial reporting. This system ensures that all patient services are accurately billed and payments are collected efficiently. It involves managing patient accounts from the initial registration through the final payment, including handling insurance claims and patient inquiries (MedStar Health, 2024). HIS can streamline these processes by integrating patient data with billing systems, thus enhancing accuracy and reducing administrative burdens (Ultimate Medical Academy, 2023).

Cost Accounting

Cost accounting in healthcare involves tracking, recording, and analyzing all costs associated with patient care and hospital operations. This includes direct costs like medical supplies and indirect costs such as administrative expenses. The goal is to determine the actual cost of services provided to help in budgeting, financial planning, and decision-making (Investopedia, 2024). HIS can provide detailed cost reports and analytics, helping administrators identify cost-saving opportunities and improve financial performance (Investopedia, 2021).

Budgeting

Budgeting in a healthcare setting involves creating a detailed financial plan that outlines expected revenues and expenses over a specific period. This process helps hospitals allocate resources efficiently, plan for future financial needs, and ensure financial stability. An administrative budget typically includes all non-production expenses such as salaries, utilities, and office supplies (Bizfluent, 2024). HIS can assist by providing real-time financial data and forecasting tools, which enhance the accuracy and efficiency of the budgeting process (Velvet Jobs, 2024).

Turnover and Absenteeism

Turnover and absenteeism are significant issues in healthcare administration, affecting both operational efficiency and patient care quality. High turnover rates can lead to increased recruitment and training costs, while absenteeism can disrupt workflow and reduce productivity. Addressing these issues involves implementing effective HR policies, providing employee support programs, and fostering a positive work environment (AIHR, 2024; Talkspace, 2024). HIS can help track and analyze employee attendance data, identify patterns, and support the development of strategies to reduce turnover and absenteeism (Randstad, 2024).

How Health Information Systems (HIS) Support Decision Making

Strategic Planning and Marketing

Health Information Systems (HIS) play a crucial role in strategic planning and marketing by providing data-driven insights that inform decision-making processes. HIS can help healthcare organizations identify market trends, patient demographics, and service utilization patterns, which are essential for developing effective marketing strategies and long-term plans. For instance, HIS can analyze patient data to identify high-demand services and target marketing efforts accordingly (Harvard Business Review, 2014). Additionally, HIS can support strategic planning by integrating data from various sources to provide a comprehensive view of the organization's performance and market position (LibreTexts, 2024).

Resource Allocation

Effective resource allocation is critical in healthcare, and HIS supports this by providing accurate and timely data on resource utilization, patient needs, and operational efficiency. HIS can track the availability and usage of medical supplies, staff, and equipment, enabling administrators to allocate resources where they are most needed (Wellcome Open Research, 2024). During the COVID-19 pandemic, for example, HIS was instrumental in managing the allocation of scarce resources such as ventilators and personal protective equipment (BMC Medical Ethics, 2022). By using HIS, healthcare organizations can ensure that resources are distributed equitably and efficiently, improving overall patient care and operational effectiveness.

Performance Evaluation and Monitoring

HIS supports performance evaluation and monitoring by providing real-time data on various performance metrics, such as patient outcomes, staff productivity, and financial performance. This data allows healthcare administrators to identify areas for improvement and implement evidence-based interventions (EvalCommunity, 2024). For example, HIS can track patient readmission rates and identify trends that may indicate issues with the quality of care. By continuously monitoring performance, healthcare organizations can make informed decisions to enhance service delivery and patient satisfaction (MEASURE Evaluation, 2019).

Product Evaluation and Services

HIS also plays a vital role in product evaluation and service improvement by collecting and analyzing data on patient experiences, treatment outcomes, and service utilization. This information helps healthcare providers assess the effectiveness of their services and identify opportunities for innovation and improvement (Harvard Business School Online, 2019). For instance, HIS can be used to gather patient feedback on new treatments or services, allowing healthcare organizations to make data-driven decisions about which products to continue, modify, or discontinue. By leveraging HIS for product evaluation, healthcare providers can ensure that they are meeting patient needs and delivering high-quality care (LibreTexts, 2024).

Evaluation and Checklist Before HIS Implementation at your organization

Capture, Storage, and Retrieval of Clinical and Financial Information

When evaluating a Health Information System (HIS), it is essential to ensure that the system can capture, store, and retrieve both clinical and financial information. This includes data related to admission, discharge, and transfer (ADT), billing, laboratory results, pharmacy records, blood bank information, and operating room schedules. Effective HIS should integrate these functionalities to streamline operations and improve data accessibility (MEASURE Evaluation, 2024).

Interface with Existing Information Systems

Another critical factor is whether the HIS can interface with your organization's existing information systems. Seamless integration is vital for ensuring data consistency and avoiding duplication of efforts. The HIS should support interoperability standards such as HL7 or FHIR to facilitate communication between different systems (Vital Strategies, 2024).

Establishing Triggers or Thresholds

The HIS should allow for the establishment of "triggers" or thresholds for important performance measures and alert administrators when these thresholds are exceeded. This feature is crucial for proactive management and timely intervention in case of deviations from expected performance (CDC, 2024).

HIS Checklist

Rule-Based Processing

- **Rule-Based Processing**: The system should have rule-based processing capabilities, meaning it can automatically generate a complete list of cases that meet or fail specific criteria. This functionality is essential for efficient case management and ensuring compliance with clinical guidelines (MEASURE Evaluation, 2024).

Flexibility for Concurrent and Retrospective Reviews

- **Flexibility**: The HIS must be flexible enough to allow both concurrent and retrospective reviews. This flexibility ensures that the system can support ongoing patient care activities as well as retrospective analyses for quality improvement and research purposes (Vital Strategies, 2024).

Support for Regulatory Requirements

- **Regulatory Compliance**: The system should support compliance with Joint Commission and other regulatory requirements. This includes features for documentation, reporting, and audit trails that meet the standards set by regulatory bodies (CDC, 2024).

Multi-User Access

- **Multi-User Access**: The HIS should allow multiple users to access the program simultaneously. This capability is crucial for ensuring that healthcare providers can collaborate effectively and access necessary information without delays (MEASURE Evaluation, 2024).

Networking Capabilities

- **Networking Capabilities**: The system should have robust networking capabilities to support data sharing and communication across different departments and locations. This feature is essential for integrated care delivery and efficient resource utilization (Vital Strategies, 2024).

2x2 Contingency Table and Predictive Value of a Test

2x2 Contingency Table

A 2x2 contingency table is a useful tool in epidemiology and diagnostic testing to evaluate the performance of a test. It categorizes test results and disease status into four possible outcomes: true positives (TP), false positives (FP), true negatives (TN), and false negatives (FN). The table is structured as follows:

	Disease Present	Disease Absent
Positive Test Result	TP	FP
Negative Test Result	FN	TN

This table helps in calculating various metrics that assess the accuracy and reliability of a diagnostic test (MedCalc, 2024).

Predictive Value of a Test

The predictive value of a test indicates the probability that a test result correctly identifies the presence or absence of a disease. There are two main types of predictive values:

Positive Predictive Value (PPV): This is the probability that a person with a positive test result actually has the disease. It is calculated using the formula:

$$PPV = \frac{TP}{TP + FP}$$

This value depends on the prevalence of the disease in the population being tested (University of Nebraska Medical Center, 2024).

Negative Predictive Value (NPV): This is the probability that a person with a negative test result does not have the disease. It is calculated using the formula:

$$NPV = \frac{TN}{FN + TN}$$

Like PPV, NPV is also influenced by the disease prevalence (University of Nebraska Medical Center, 2024).

Sensitivity and Specificity in Diagnostic Testing

Sensitivity

Sensitivity, also known as the True Positive Rate (TPR), measures the ability of a test to correctly identify individuals who have the disease. It is calculated using the formula:

$$TPR = \frac{TP}{FN + TP}$$

where (TP) represents true positives and (FN) represents false negatives. A high sensitivity indicates that the test is effective in detecting the disease among those who are truly diseased (MedCalc, 2024). For example, if a test has a sensitivity of 99.9%, it means that 99.9% of the individuals with the disease are correctly identified by the test.

Specificity

Specificity, also known as the True Negative Rate (TNR), measures the ability of a test to correctly identify individuals who do not have the disease. It is calculated using the formula:

$$TNR = \frac{TN}{FP + TN}$$

where (TN) represents true negatives and (FP) represents false positives. A high specificity indicates that the test is effective in identifying healthy individuals who do not have the disease (IBM, 2024). For instance, a test with a specificity of 99.9% means that 99.9% of the individuals without the disease are correctly identified as disease-free.

False Negative Rate and False Positive Rate

False Negative Rate

The False Negative Rate (FNR) is a measure used to evaluate the performance of a diagnostic test. It represents the proportion of individuals with the disease who are incorrectly identified as not having the disease. The FNR is calculated as:

FNR=1−Sensitivity

where Sensitivity (or True Positive Rate) is the ability of the test to correctly identify those with the disease (MedCalc, 2024). For example, if a test has a sensitivity of 95%, the FNR would be:

FNR=1−0.95=0.05 or 5%

This means that 5% of the individuals with the disease are not detected by the test.

False Positive Rate

The False Positive Rate (FPR) is another important measure in diagnostic testing. It indicates the proportion of individuals without the disease who are incorrectly identified as having the disease. The FPR is calculated as:

FPR=1−Specificity

where Specificity (or True Negative Rate) is the ability of the test to correctly identify those without the disease (IBM, 2024). For instance, if a test has a specificity of 99%, the FPR would be:

FPR=1−0.99=0.01 or 1%

This implies that 1% of the individuals without the disease are incorrectly identified as having the disease.

Input Devices

Keyboard

A keyboard is one of the most common input devices used to enter data into a computer. It consists of a set of keys that include letters, numbers, and various function keys. Keyboards are essential for typing text and executing commands (Javatpoint, 2024).

Menu/Cursor

Menu and cursor input devices allow users to interact with graphical user interfaces (GUIs). These devices include pointing devices like a mouse, which moves the cursor on the screen to select items from menus or execute commands (KnowComputing, 2024).

Graphical User Interface (GUI)

Graphical User Interfaces (GUIs) use devices such as a mouse, touch screen, and light pen to facilitate user interaction with the computer. A mouse is a pointing device that allows users to move a cursor and select objects on the screen. Touch screens enable direct interaction with the display by touching it, while light pens allow users to draw or select items directly on the screen (CHTips, 2024).

Voice Recognition

Voice recognition systems convert spoken words into digital data. These systems are used for hands-free computing and accessibility, allowing users to control devices and input data using their voice (Javatpoint, 2024).

Optical Character Recognition (OCR)

Optical Character Recognition (OCR) is a technology that converts different types of documents, such as scanned paper documents or PDFs, into editable and searchable data. OCR systems scan the text and convert it into machine-readable code (KnowComputing, 2024).

CPU

Central Processing Unit (CPU)

The Central Processing Unit (CPU) is the primary component of a computer that performs most of the processing inside a computer. It executes instructions from programs and coordinates the activities of all other hardware components (Total Phase, 2023).

Registers (16, 32, or 64 bit)

Registers are small, fast storage locations within the CPU that hold data and instructions temporarily. They come in various sizes, such as 16-bit, 32-bit, and 64-bit, which determine the amount of data they can handle at one time. Larger registers can process more data and perform more complex calculations (Total Phase, 2023).

Operating Speed

The operating speed of a CPU, often measured in gigahertz (GHz), indicates how many cycles per second it can execute. Higher operating speeds generally mean faster processing and better performance (Computer Info Bits, 2024).

RAM

Random Access Memory (RAM) is a type of computer memory that is used to store data and machine code currently being used. RAM is much faster than other types of storage, such as hard drives, and is crucial for the efficient operation of the CPU (Learn Computer Science Online, 2024).

Memory and Storage

RAM: Data is Deleted When PC is Shut Off

Random Access Memory (RAM) is a type of volatile memory used to store data that is actively being used or processed by the computer. The data in RAM is lost when the computer is turned off or restarted, making it temporary storage. RAM is essential for the smooth operation of applications and the operating system, as it allows for quick read and write access to a large amount of data (Telnyx, 2024).

ROM: Data is Permanent

Read-Only Memory (ROM) is non-volatile memory that permanently stores data. Unlike RAM, the data in ROM is not lost when the computer is powered off. ROM is typically used to store firmware, which is the software that is permanently programmed into the hardware. This includes the system's BIOS (Basic Input/Output System), which is essential for booting up the computer and performing hardware initialization during the startup process (Telnyx, 2024).

Active Storage

Active storage refers to storage systems that are actively used for data processing and retrieval. This includes primary storage devices like RAM and secondary storage devices such as hard drives and solid-state drives (SSDs). Active storage is crucial for the day-to-day operations of a computer system, as it provides the necessary space for running applications and accessing frequently used data (1Gbits, 2024).

Archival Storage

Archival storage is used for long-term data preservation and is typically not accessed frequently. This type of storage is essential for maintaining historical records, backups, and compliance with data retention policies. Archival storage solutions include magnetic tapes, optical discs, and cloud storage services. These systems are designed to be cost-effective and durable, ensuring that data remains intact and accessible over extended periods (Save My Exams, 2024).

Optical Storage

Optical storage uses lasers to read and write data on discs made of plastic with a reflective coating. Common types of optical storage include CDs (Compact Discs), DVDs (Digital Versatile Discs), and Blu-ray discs. Data is encoded in the form of tiny pits and lands on the surface of the disc, which are interpreted by the laser. Optical storage is non-volatile, meaning it retains data even when the power is off. It is often used for media distribution, backups, and archival purposes due to its durability and portability (1Gbits, 2024).

Computer Architecture

Mainframe

Mainframes are powerful computers used primarily by large organizations for critical applications, bulk data processing, and large-scale transaction processing. They are known for their high reliability, availability, and serviceability (RAS). Mainframes can handle vast amounts of data and support thousands of users simultaneously. For example, IBM's zSeries mainframes are used by major banks and airlines to process millions of transactions per second (IBM, 2024).

Server

Servers are computers designed to manage network resources and provide services to other computers, known as clients. They can handle multiple tasks simultaneously and are essential for hosting websites, managing databases, and running applications. Servers vary in size and capacity, from small home servers to large enterprise servers. For instance, a web server hosts websites and delivers web pages to users' browsers (Microsoft, 2024).

Workstation

Workstations are high-performance computers designed for technical or scientific applications. They offer greater performance than personal computers (PCs) and are used for tasks such as 3D rendering, complex calculations, and software development. Workstations typically have powerful processors, large amounts of RAM, and high-end graphics capabilities. An example is the Dell Precision series, which is used by engineers and designers for CAD (Computer-Aided Design) applications (Dell, 2024).

PC (Personal Computer)

Personal computers (PCs) are general-purpose computers designed for individual use. They are versatile and can be used for a wide range of tasks, including word processing, internet browsing, gaming, and multimedia. PCs come in various forms, such as desktops, laptops, and tablets. An example is the HP Pavilion series, which is popular among home users for its balance of performance and affordability (HP, 2024).

Terminal

Terminals are devices used to interact with mainframes or servers. They do not perform any processing themselves but rely on the central computer for processing power. Terminals can be simple text-based devices or more advanced graphical terminals. Historically, terminals were used to access mainframe computers in large organizations. Modern equivalents include thin clients, which are used in environments where centralized computing is preferred (Citrix, 2024).

Differences Between Computer Architectures

- **Mainframes vs. Servers**: Mainframes are designed for high-volume transaction processing and can support thousands of users simultaneously, whereas servers are more versatile and can be used for a variety of network services. Mainframes are typically used in large enterprises, while servers are used in both small and large organizations (IBM, 2024; Microsoft, 2024).
- **Workstations vs. PCs**: Workstations offer higher performance and are used for specialized tasks requiring significant computational power, such as 3D rendering and scientific simulations. PCs are more general-purpose and are used for everyday tasks by individuals (Dell, 2024; HP, 2024).
- **Terminals vs. PCs**: Terminals rely on a central computer for processing and are used in environments where centralized control is needed. PCs are standalone devices that perform all processing locally

and are used for a wide range of personal and professional tasks (Citrix, 2024).

Computerized Physician Order Entry (CPOE)

Implementation of CPOE

Computerized Physician Order Entry (CPOE) systems were first implemented in the United States in the 1970s, with significant adoption occurring in the 1990s and 2000s as part of broader efforts to improve healthcare quality and reduce errors (Sittig & Stead, 1994). In Saudi Arabia, CPOE implementation began more recently, with notable projects starting in the early 2000s. For instance, the National Guard Health Affairs (NGHA) in Riyadh implemented CPOE to enhance patient safety and reduce medication errors (Altuwaijri, 2008).

Examples of Savings in Healthcare Systems

United States

In Massachusetts, the implementation of CPOE systems has led to substantial financial savings. A study estimated that CPOE could save approximately $140.7 million annually by reducing medication errors, improving efficiency, and decreasing adverse drug events (Bates et al., 1999). These savings are attributed to the reduction in costs associated with correcting medication errors and the improved workflow efficiency that CPOE systems provide.

Saudi Arabia

In Saudi Arabia, the implementation of CPOE at the National Guard Health Affairs (NGHA) has also demonstrated significant benefits. The system has improved patient safety by reducing medication errors and enhancing the efficiency of clinical workflows. Although specific financial savings figures are not widely published, the qualitative benefits include better resource utilization and improved patient outcomes (Altuwaijri, 2008).

e-Health and Telemedicine

Telemedicine

Telemedicine involves the use of medical information exchanged from one site to another via electronic communications to improve a patient's health status. This practice allows healthcare providers to diagnose, treat, and monitor patients remotely, enhancing access to medical services, especially in underserved areas (World Health Organization, 2024).

Telemedicine Services

Telemedicine encompasses a variety of services across different medical specialties:

- **Radiology**: Remote interpretation of medical images such as X-rays, CT scans, and MRIs.
- **Dermatology**: Diagnosis and treatment of skin conditions through digital images and video consultations.
- **Ophthalmology**: Eye examinations and consultations conducted remotely.
- **Pathology**: Analysis of laboratory samples and pathology reports via digital platforms.
- **Cardiology**: Remote monitoring and consultation for heart-related conditions.
- **Psychiatry**: Mental health services provided through video conferencing and other digital means (Telemedicine and e-Health, 2024).

Telemedicine Services

Telemedicine offers several key services:

- **Specialist Referral Services**: Enables primary care providers to consult with specialists remotely.
- **Patient Consultations**: Direct consultations between patients and healthcare providers via video calls.

- **Remote Patient Monitoring**: Continuous monitoring of patients' health data using wearable devices and sensors.
- **Medical Education**: Training and continuing education for healthcare professionals through online platforms (Anthony, 2021).

Telemedicine Mechanisms

Telemedicine can be delivered through two primary mechanisms:

- **Synchronous**: Real-time, full-motion video and audio communication between patients and healthcare providers. This method requires more bandwidth and is used for live consultations and immediate feedback (Anthony, 2021).
- **Asynchronous**: Also known as "store-and-forward," this method involves transmitting medical data to a healthcare provider for review at a later time. It requires less bandwidth and allows clinicians to access information at their convenience (Telemedicine and e-Health, 2024).

e-Health Clinical Applications

e-Health encompasses various clinical applications that enhance patient care:

- **Rx Renewals**: Electronic prescription renewals.
- **Test Results**: Online access to laboratory and diagnostic test results.
- **Self-Monitoring Status**: Tools for patients to monitor their health conditions at home.
- **Non-Urgent e-Consults**: Electronic consultations for non-emergency medical issues.
- **Uploading Data from Home Monitoring Devices with Clinical Feedback**: Integration of data from home monitoring devices into the patient's electronic health record, with feedback from healthcare providers (Telemedicine and e-Health, 2024).

e-Health Administrative Applications

e-Health also includes administrative applications that streamline healthcare operations:

- **Appointment Requests**: Online scheduling of medical appointments.
- **Update Information**: Patients can update their personal and medical information online.
- **Online Bill Payment**: Electronic payment of medical bills.
- **Non-Clinical Patient Inquiries**: Handling of administrative questions and concerns through digital platforms (Anthony, 2021).

References:

1. Altuwaijri, M. M. (2008). Implementation of Computerized Physician Order Entry (CPOE) towards Patient Safety in Saudi Hospitals. Bulletin of High Institute of Public Health, 38(2), 459-470. https://jhiphalexu.journals.ekb.eg/article_20898_af04f62a156b33eb5594bd82038dffc3.pdf

2. American Institute for Healthcare Management. (2024). Healthcare Data Quality. https://www.amihm.org/healthcare-data-quality/

3. American Medical Association. (2012). Electronic Health Records: Privacy, Confidentiality, and Security. https://journalofethics.ama-assn.org/article/electronic-health-records-privacy-confidentiality-and-security/2012-09

4. Anthony, J. (2021). Application of telemedicine and eHealth technology for clinical services in response to COVID-19 pandemic. Health and Technology, 11, 359–366. https://link.springer.com/article/10.1007/s12553-020-00516-4

5. Bates, D. W., et al. (1999). Effect of computerized physician order entry and a team intervention on prevention of serious medication errors. JAMA, 280(15), 1311-1316.

6. Boonstra, A., & Broekhuis, M. (2010). Barriers to the acceptance of electronic medical records by physicians from systematic review to taxonomy and interventions. BMC Health Services Research, 10, 231. https://bmchealthservres.biomedcentral.com/articles/10.1186/1472-6963-10-231

7. Brown, A. (2022). User-centered design in healthcare IT. Journal of Healthcare Information Management, 36(4), 45-58.

8. Calysta EMR. (2023). Overcoming barriers: Encouraging physician adoption of electronic health record systems. https://calystaemr.com/physician-adoption-of-electronic-health-record-systems/

9. CAQH. (2023). Breaking down barriers: The impact of HER integrations on healthcare efficiency and care delivery. https://www.caqh.org/blog/breaking-down-barriers-impact-ehr-integrations-healthcare-efficiency-and-care-delivery

10. Centers for Disease Control and Prevention (CDC). (2024). Good evaluation questions: A checklist to help focus your evaluation. https://www.cdc.gov/evaluation/pdf/CDC_Eval_Framework_Checklist.pdf

11. CMS. (2024). Electronic health records.
    https://www.cms.gov/priorities/key-initiatives/e-health/records

12. DesHarnais, S., Moore, F. D., & Kazandjian, V. A. (2023). Hospital readmissions as a measure of quality of health care: Advantages and limitations. JAMA Internal Medicine.

13. Hebda, T., & Czar, P. (2013). Handbook of informatics for nurses and healthcare professionals. Pearson.

14. HealthIT.gov. (2024). What are electronic health records (EHRs)?
    https://www.healthit.gov/topic/health-it-and-health-information-exchange-basics/what-are-electronic-health-records-ehrs

15. Holmgren, A. J., McBride, S., Gale, B., & Mossburg, S. (2023). Technology as a tool for improving patient safety. PSNet.
    https://psnet.ahrq.gov/perspective/technology-tool-improving-patient-safety

16. Holmgren, A. J., McBride, S., Gale, B., & Mossburg, S. (2023). Technology as a tool for improving patient safety. PSNet.
    https://psnet.ahrq.gov/perspective/technology-tool-improving-patient-safety

17. Johnson, M. (2021). The role of IT in healthcare business processes. Healthcare Management Review, 34(2), 123-135.

18. Langate. (2023). EMR Integration: Ultimate Guide.
    https://langate.com/emr-integration-ultimate-guide/

19. Mainz, J. (2003). Defining and classifying clinical indicators for quality improvement. International Journal for Quality in Health Care, 15(6), 523-530.

20. McGonigle, D., & Mastrian, K. G. (2021). Nursing informatics and the foundation of knowledge. Jones & Bartlett Learning.

21. MEASURE Evaluation. (2024). HIS Assessment Tools.
    https://www.measureevaluation.org/his-strengthening-resource-center/his-assessment-tools.html

22. National Center for Health Statistics. (2012). National perceptions of HER adoption: Barriers, impacts, and federal policies.
    https://www.cdc.gov/nchs/ppt/nchs2012/ss-03_jamoom.pdf

23. SelectHub. (2024). HER implementation cost breakdown in 2024.
    https://www.selecthub.com/medical-software/ehr-implementation-cost/

24. Sittig, D. F., & Stead, W. W. (1994). Computer-based physician order entry: the state of the art. Journal of the American Medical Informatics Association, 1(2), 108-123.

25. Smith, T., & Jones, L. (2023). IT as a support service in healthcare. International Journal of Medical Informatics, 45(1), 67-79.

26. Tan, J. K. H., & Payton, F. C. (2010). Adaptive health management information systems: Concepts, cases, & practical applications. Jones & Bartlett Learning.

27. USF Health Online. (2024). What are electronic medical records (EMRs)? https://www.usfhealthonline.com/resources/health-informatics/what-are-electronic-medical-records-emr/

28. U.S. Department of Health and Human Services. (2024). Summary of the HIPAA Privacy Rule. https://www.hhs.gov/hipaa/for-professionals/privacy/laws-regulations/index.html

29. Wager, K. A., Lee, F. W., & Glaser, J. P. (2017). Health care information systems: A practical approach for health care management. Jossey-Bass.

30. World Health Organization. (2024). Telemedicine: Opportunities and developments in Member States. https://www.who.int/goe/publications/goe_telemedicine_2010.pdf

31. Yasnoff, W. A., et al. (2001). Public health informatics: Improving and transforming public health in the information age. Journal of Public Health Management and Practice, 7(6), 67-75.

32. Zook, C. J., & Moore, F. D. (1980). High cost users of medical care. New England Journal of Medicine, 302(996-1002).

Chapter 14

Healthcare Risk Management

Omar Ibn Al-Khattab, the second Caliph of the Islamic Empire, stated: "If a mule stumbled in Iraq, I would be responsible for it before God for not having paved the way for it."

The capital of the empire was in Al-Madinah Al-Munawarah (western Saudi Arabia). As a leader, he took full accountability not only for the safety of human beings, but also for a mule living 1500 kilometers away from the capital. This quote shows that the concepts of safety, risk, and accountability management evolved and were applied over 15 centuries ago.

Risk and Hazard Defined:

Risk refers to the uncertainty about future events that may threaten the safety of patients, as well as the assets and reputations of healthcare providers. This concept encompasses various types of risks, including clinical, operational, financial, and strategic risks (HIPAA Journal, 2024). Clinical risks involve potential harm to patients due to medical errors, infections, or other adverse events. For example, medication errors and surgical mistakes are common clinical risks that healthcare providers must manage (Riskonnect, 2024). Operational risks pertain to the internal processes and systems within healthcare organizations. These risks can arise from human errors, system failures, or inadequate procedures, potentially leading to disruptions in healthcare delivery (HIPAA Journal, 2024).

Financial risks in healthcare include the potential for financial losses due to fraud, malpractice lawsuits, or regulatory fines. These risks can significantly impact the financial stability of healthcare organizations (Riskonnect, 2024). Strategic risks are associated with the broader goals and direction of the organization, such as adapting to new technologies or regulatory changes. Failure to manage these risks can result in reputational damage and loss of competitive advantage (HIPAA Journal, 2024).

It is an organized effort to identify, assess, and reduce risks to patients, staff, visitors, and assets (HIPAA Journal, 2024).

Identify: The first step in risk management is to identify potential risks. This includes recognizing hazards that could cause harm to patients, staff, visitors, or assets. For example, identifying risks such as medication errors, equipment failures, or security breaches is crucial (Riskonnect, 2024).

Assess: Once risks are identified, the next step is to assess their likelihood and potential impact. This involves evaluating the probability of occurrence and the severity of the consequences if the risk materializes. For instance, assessing the risk of a data breach would involve understanding both the likelihood of such an event and the potential damage to patient privacy and organizational reputation (HIPAA Journal, 2024).

Reduce: The final step is to implement measures to reduce or mitigate the identified risks. This can include a variety of strategies such as training staff, improving procedures, investing in better equipment, or enhancing security protocols. The goal is to minimize the likelihood of risks occurring and to lessen their impact if they do (Riskonnect, 2024).

A hazard, on the other hand, is defined as a situation, condition, or object that has the potential to cause harm, loss, or damage to life, health, property, or the environment (The Knowledge Academy, 2024). Hazards can be categorized into different types, such as physical (e.g., earthquakes, floods), chemical (e.g., toxic substances, explosives), biological (e.g., pathogens, allergens), ergonomic (e.g., repetitive strain, poor posture), and psychosocial (e.g., stress, violence) (The Knowledge Academy, 2024). The severity and likelihood of the harm that a hazard can cause vary widely, depending on factors such as the nature of the hazard, the environment in which it occurs, and the vulnerability of those exposed to it (Worksafe UK, 2024).

The key difference between risk and hazard lies in their definitions and focus. Risk refers to the possibility of experiencing harm, loss, or adverse effects resulting from exposure to hazards. It quantifies the likelihood and potential severity of adverse outcomes arising from a particular situation or action (The Knowledge Academy, 2024). In contrast, a hazard is a potential source of harm, focusing on identifying what could cause harm without considering the likelihood of occurrence (Worksafe UK, 2024). Risk involves assessing how likely it is that the hazard will lead to harm and how severe that harm would be, while hazard management aims to eliminate, reduce, or control the hazard itself to prevent potential harm (The Knowledge Academy, 2024).

Assets in Healthcare:

- **People:** This category includes patients, clinicians, volunteers, and employees. These individuals are essential to the functioning of healthcare organizations and their safety and well-being are paramount (Fracttal, 2023).
- **Property:** This encompasses buildings, facilities, equipment, and materials. These physical assets are necessary for providing healthcare services and maintaining operational efficiency (Revnue, 2025).
- **Financial:** Financial assets include revenue, reserves, grants, and reimbursement. These resources are crucial for the financial stability and sustainability of healthcare organizations (About Financials, 2024).
- **Goodwill:** Goodwill refers to the health and well-being reputation and stature in the community. This intangible asset is vital for maintaining trust and credibility with patients and the broader community (Fracttal, 2023).

Objective of Risk Management:

- **To reduce the risk of preventable accidents and injuries:** This involves implementing measures to prevent incidents such as medical errors, equipment failures, and other hazards that could harm patients, staff, or visitors (Berxi, 2024).
- **To minimize financial loss if one occurs:** Effective risk management strategies help healthcare organizations mitigate the financial impact of adverse events, such as malpractice lawsuits, regulatory fines, and other financial liabilities (HIPAA Journal, 2024).

Risk management provides strategies, techniques, and approaches to recognizing and confronting any threat faced by an organization. These strategies include developing comprehensive risk management plans, conducting regular risk assessments, and implementing preventive measures to address identified risks (ASHRM, 2024).

Risk Model

Risk = Probability x Impact

This formula helps quantify the potential risk by considering both the likelihood of an event occurring and the severity of its consequences (HIPAA Journal, 2024).

Example: Reducing the Risk of a Young Boy Falling Off His Bike

To illustrate this model, consider the scenario of reducing the risk of a young boy falling off his bike. The risk can be managed by addressing both the probability of the event occurring and the impact if it does occur.

Reduce Probability (Chances):

Teaching the boy how to ride a bike: By providing proper training, the likelihood of falling decreases as the boy becomes more skilled and confident in riding.

Forbidding him from riding it: This eliminates the risk entirely by removing the activity that could lead to a fall (Riskonnect, 2024).

Reduce Impact (Severity):

Using a helmet: This reduces the severity of injury if a fall occurs, protecting the boy's head.

Adding two wheels (training wheels): This stabilizes the bike, making it less likely for the boy to fall and thus reducing the potential impact of a fall (Berxi, 2024).

Risk Manager:

A risk manager in healthcare is a crucial asset to any facility, responsible for identifying, evaluating, and applying risk management techniques to mitigate potential threats. This role involves a variety of responsibilities and duties that are essential for maintaining patient safety and organizational stability.

Responsibilities of a Risk Manager:

- **Risk Identification:** The risk manager is tasked with identifying potential risks that could affect patients, staff, visitors, and the organization's assets. This includes recognizing hazards such as medical errors, equipment failures, and security breaches (HIPAA Journal, 2024).
- **Risk Evaluation:** Once risks are identified, the risk manager evaluates their likelihood and potential impact. This involves assessing the probability of occurrence and the severity of consequences if the risk materializes (Riskonnect, 2024).
- **Application of Risk Management Techniques:** The risk manager applies various techniques to manage and mitigate risks. This includes implementing policies and procedures, training staff, and developing risk management plans. One key technique is risk shifting, which involves transferring the risk to another party, such as through insurance (ASHRM, 2024).

Duties of a Risk Manager:

The duties of a risk manager can vary widely but generally include performing basic risk management functions such as:

- **Developing and Implementing Risk Management Plans:** Creating comprehensive plans to address identified risks and ensure they are managed effectively (HealthcareDegree.com, 2024).
- **Conducting Risk Assessments:** Regularly assessing risks to identify new threats and evaluate the effectiveness of existing risk management strategies (ASHRM, 2024).
- **Training Staff:** Educating employees on risk management practices and how to recognize and avoid potential risks (InterviewGuy, 2024).
- **Monitoring and Reporting:** Continuously monitoring risk management activities and reporting on their effectiveness to senior management (HealthcareDegree.com, 2024).

Risk Management process:

Risk management in healthcare involves several key steps, often summarized by the three R's and five I's.

Three R's:

- **Risk Identification:** This step involves recognizing potential risks that could affect patients, staff, visitors, or the organization's assets. For example, identifying risks such as medication errors, equipment failures, or security breaches is crucial (HIPAA Journal, 2024).
- **Risk Analysis:** Once risks are identified, they must be analyzed to determine their likelihood and potential impact. This involves assessing the probability of occurrence and the severity of consequences if the risk materializes (Riskonnect, 2024).
- **Risk Control/Treatment:** The final step is to implement measures to control or treat the identified risks. This can include a variety of strategies such as training staff, improving procedures, investing in better equipment, or enhancing security protocols (Berxi, 2024).

Five I's:

- **Investigate:** This involves thoroughly examining the identified risks to understand their root causes and potential effects (ASHRM, 2024).
- **Inform:** Communicating the identified risks and their potential impacts to relevant stakeholders is essential. This ensures that everyone involved is aware of the risks and the measures being taken to address them (HealthcareDegree.com, 2024).
- **Influence:** This step involves advocating for necessary changes and influencing decision-makers to implement risk management strategies (InterviewGuy, 2024).
- **Interpret:** Analyzing data and interpreting the results to make informed decisions about risk management strategies (ASHRM, 2024).
- **Integrate:** Integrating risk management practices into the organization's overall operations to ensure a cohesive approach to managing risks (HealthcareDegree.com, 2024).

Risk Plan

Healthcare organizations typically have a risk management plan that outlines their philosophy and approach to managing risks. Often, this plan is integrated with the quality management plan due to the interconnected nature of these processes (Berxi, 2024).

Components of a Risk Plan:

- **Plan:** A detailed document that describes the risk management strategies and procedures specific to the organization. This includes the identification, assessment, and mitigation of risks (HIPAA Journal, 2024).
- **Board Statement Support of Risk Management:** A formal statement from the organization's board of directors endorsing the risk management plan and its importance. This demonstrates top-level commitment to managing risks effectively (Berxi, 2024).

- **Confidentiality Assertions:** Policies and procedures to ensure that sensitive information related to risk management is kept confidential. This includes protecting patient data and other proprietary information (SafetyCulture, 2023).
- **Data Collection and Reporting Mechanism:** Systems for collecting and reporting data on risks, both internally and externally. This includes mechanisms for tracking incidents, analyzing trends, and reporting findings to relevant stakeholders (AlertMedia, 2023).
- **Integration with Quality Management:** Ensuring that risk management activities are aligned with quality management processes to enhance overall organizational performance. This integration helps in identifying and addressing risks that could impact the quality of care (Berxi, 2024).
- **Program Effectiveness Reviews:** Regular reviews of the risk management program to assess its effectiveness and make necessary improvements. This involves evaluating the outcomes of risk management activities and adjusting strategies as needed (HIPAA Journal, 2024).

Risk Management planning tools:

Risk management planning in healthcare involves various tools and techniques to effectively identify, assess, and mitigate risks. Here are some key tools used in the process:

Meetings:
- Regular meetings are essential for discussing potential risks, reviewing incidents, and planning risk management strategies. These meetings facilitate communication and collaboration among different departments and stakeholders (ASHRM, 2024).

Documentation Review:
- Reviewing existing documentation, such as policies, procedures, incident reports, and audit findings, helps identify areas of risk and opportunities for improvement. This process ensures that all relevant information is considered in the risk management plan (HIPAA Journal, 2024).

Information Gathering:

- **Brainstorming:** This technique involves gathering a group of stakeholders to generate ideas and identify potential risks through open discussion. Brainstorming sessions can uncover risks that might not be immediately obvious (Riskonnect, 2024).
- **Delphi Technique:** This method uses a series of questionnaires to gather input from experts. The responses are aggregated and shared with the group, and the process is repeated until a consensus is reached. This technique is useful for obtaining expert opinions on complex risks (Berxi, 2024).
- **Interviews:** Conducting interviews with staff, patients, and other stakeholders provides valuable insights into potential risks and areas for improvement. Interviews can reveal firsthand experiences and concerns that might not be captured through other methods (ASHRM, 2024).

Risk Management and Activities

Risk management in healthcare involves a variety of activities and functions aimed at identifying, assessing, and mitigating risks to ensure patient safety and organizational stability. Here are some key activities and functions of risk management:

Risk Acceptance: This involves acknowledging the presence of a risk and deciding to accept it without taking any action to mitigate it. This is typically done when the cost of mitigating the risk is higher than the potential impact of the risk itself (HIPAA Journal, 2024).

Exposure Avoidance: This strategy involves taking steps to avoid exposure to certain risks altogether. For example, a healthcare facility might avoid using certain high-risk procedures or equipment to eliminate the associated risks (Riskonnect, 2024).

Loss Prevention: This involves implementing measures to prevent losses from occurring. For instance, regular maintenance of medical equipment can prevent malfunctions that could lead to patient harm (Berxi, 2024).

Loss Reduction: This strategy focuses on reducing the severity of losses when they occur. For example, using protective gear like helmets and gloves can reduce the impact of falls or other accidents (ASHRM, 2024).

Exposure Segregation: This involves separating high-risk activities or areas from other parts of the organization to contain potential risks. For example, isolating infectious patients in a separate ward to prevent the spread of disease (SafetyCulture, 2023).

Contractual Transfer: This involves transferring risk to another party through contracts, such as purchasing insurance to cover potential financial losses (HIPAA Journal, 2024).

Risk Financing: This involves securing funds to cover potential losses. This can include purchasing insurance or setting aside reserves to cover unexpected costs (Riskonnect, 2024).

Incident Identification, Reporting, and Tracking: This involves identifying and documenting incidents that occur, reporting them to relevant authorities, and tracking them to identify patterns and prevent recurrence (Berxi, 2024).

Incident Review and Evaluation: This involves reviewing and evaluating incidents to understand their causes and impacts, and to develop strategies to prevent similar incidents in the future (ASHRM, 2024).

Actions to Prevent Recurrence of Incidents: Implementing corrective actions based on incident reviews to prevent similar incidents from happening again (SafetyCulture, 2023).

Internal Documentation: Maintaining detailed records of risk management activities, incidents, and corrective actions to ensure accountability and continuous improvement (HIPAA Journal, 2024).

Education: Providing training and education to staff on risk management practices and procedures to ensure they are aware of potential risks and how to mitigate them (Riskonnect, 2024).

Liaison with Regulators, Insurers, etc.: Working with regulatory bodies, insurers, and other external stakeholders to ensure compliance with regulations and to secure necessary support and resources (ASHRM, 2024).

Managing Liabilities: Identifying and managing potential liabilities to protect the organization from legal and financial repercussions (Berxi, 2024).

Risk Management Resources:

- **The Risk Manager:** The individual responsible for overseeing the risk management program, identifying potential risks, and implementing strategies to mitigate them (ASHRM, 2024).
- **RM Coordinators:** Staff members who assist the risk manager in executing risk management activities, ensuring compliance with risk management policies across departments (Riskonnect, 2024).
- **Organizational Structure:** The framework within which risk management activities are organized, including the hierarchy and reporting lines (ASHRM, 2024).
- **Roles and Responsibilities:** Clearly defined roles and responsibilities for all staff involved in risk management to ensure accountability and effective implementation of risk management strategies (Berxi, 2024).
- **RM Committee:** A dedicated committee that oversees risk management activities, reviews risk assessments, and makes recommendations for improvement (ASHRM, 2024).
- **Outsourcing Functions:** Engaging external experts or organizations to handle specific risk management functions, such as conducting audits or providing specialized training (SafetyCulture, 2023).

Risk Management Sources:

- **Documentation Review and Audit:** Reviewing existing documents and conducting audits to identify potential risks and areas for improvement. This process helps ensure that all relevant information is considered in the risk management plan (Carroll, 2019).

- **Peer Review:** Evaluating the performance and practices of peers to identify risks and ensure compliance with standards. Peer review is a critical component of maintaining high standards in healthcare (Youngberg, 2011).
- **Incident Report:** Collecting and analyzing reports of incidents to identify patterns and prevent recurrence. Incident reporting systems are essential for tracking and addressing adverse events (ECRI Institute, 2020).
- **Infection Control Data:** Monitoring infection control data to identify and mitigate risks related to infections. Effective infection control practices are crucial for patient safety (Pittet, Allegranzi, & Storr, 2008).
- **Self-Assessment:** Conducting self-assessments to identify risks and evaluate the effectiveness of risk management practices. Self-assessment tools help organizations proactively identify and address potential issues (Reason, 2016).
- **Proactive Approach:** Implementing proactive measures to identify and mitigate risks before they occur. This includes strategies such as failure mode and effects analysis (FMEA) (Vincent, 2010).
- **Key Performance Indicators Data:** Using data from key performance indicators to monitor and manage risks. KPIs provide measurable insights into the effectiveness of risk management strategies (Griffith, 2020).
- **Complaints:** Analyzing complaints from patients, staff, and other stakeholders to identify and address potential risks. Complaints can provide valuable feedback for improving safety and quality (Leape, 1994).
- **Others:** Other sources of risk information can include regulatory guidelines, industry best practices, and feedback from external audits. These sources help ensure compliance and continuous improvement (Carroll, 2019).

Organizational Structure and Risk Management:

In healthcare organizations, the risk management unit may report directly to the medical director or, in some cases, to the chief executive officer

(CEO). This reporting structure ensures that risk management activities are aligned with the organization's overall strategic goals and receive the necessary support from top leadership (Ferdosi, Rezayatmand, & Molavi Taleghani, 2020).

Risk Management Committee:

The risk management unit is supported by a multifunctional or multidisciplinary team of professionals representing the most relevant functions and departments within the organization. This committee is typically chaired by the risk manager and assisted by one or two coordinators. The Quality Assurance (QA) coordinator is also a key member of this committee. The committee's role is to oversee risk management activities, review risk assessments, and develop strategies to mitigate identified risks (Niv & Tal, 2023).

Outsourcing Risk Management:

In smaller healthcare organizations, certain tasks or activities related to risk management may be delegated or outsourced to external organizations. This can include functions such as compliance audits, staff training, and risk assessments. Outsourcing allows smaller organizations to leverage external expertise and resources, ensuring that risk management activities are conducted effectively without overburdening internal staff (Ferdosi et al., 2020).

Costs of Risks

Appraisal Costs

Appraisal costs are associated with activities that ensure quality and compliance within an organization. These include costs related to surveying, problem solving, auditing, inspecting, peer reviews, utilization management, preparing for accreditation, and risk management. According to Jensen et al. (2022), risk assessment matrices are a practical tool for characterizing hazard risk by accounting for severity and likelihood, which is essential for effective risk management (Jensen et al., 2022).

Prevention Costs

Prevention costs are incurred to prevent problems before they occur. These costs include training, education, awareness activities, preventive management, and preventive maintenance. For instance, implementing educational programs for handling specialized equipment can significantly reduce risks (Swisher et al., 2004). The cost-benefit analysis of prevention programs often shows that they are cost-effective, with savings per dollar spent ranging from $2.00 to $19.64 (Swisher et al., 2004).

Internal Failure Costs

Internal failure costs arise from errors that occur within the organization but do not directly affect the patient or customer. These include costs associated with duplications of procedures or rework. Poor risk management can lead to significant internal failure costs, as highlighted by Ferede et al. (2020), who noted that these costs often stem from inefficiencies in processes and the need for rework (Ferede et al., 2020).

External Failure Costs

External failure costs are incurred when errors affect the patient or customer, leading to varying degrees of severity and impact. These costs can include malpractice, medical errors, and other significant failures. Kaplan and Mikes (2016) discuss how effective risk management can mitigate these costs by identifying and addressing risks early, thus preventing severe consequences (Kaplan & Mikes, 2016).

Risk Management from the Donabedian Model Perspective

Managing Structural Risks

Human Resources Training and education of staff and patients are crucial for increasing awareness of potential risks within an organization and for learning ways to avoid or control these risks. According to Grol and Grimshaw (2003), continuous professional development and training programs are essential for maintaining high standards of care and minimizing risks (Grol & Grimshaw, 2003).

Physical Resources Managing physical resources involves scheduling periodic preventive maintenance of all equipment, posting signs of caution, updating old equipment, and ensuring effective calibration of machines. As noted by Reason (2000), regular maintenance and updates are critical for preventing equipment failures and ensuring patient safety (Reason, 2000).

Managing Process Risks

Clinical Practice Guidelines Clinical practice guidelines help standardize care and reduce variability, which can minimize risks. Woolf et al. (1999) emphasize that adherence to well-developed guidelines can improve patient outcomes and reduce errors (Woolf et al., 1999).

Policies and Procedures Establishing clear policies and procedures is fundamental for risk management. These documents provide a framework for consistent practice and decision-making, which is essential for minimizing risks (Kaplan & Mikes, 2016).

Critical Pathways Critical pathways are structured multidisciplinary care plans that detail essential steps in the care of patients with specific clinical problems. They are designed to reduce variability in clinical practice and improve outcomes (Rotter et al., 2010).

Accreditation Standards Accreditation standards ensure that healthcare organizations meet specific performance criteria, which can help manage risks by promoting high-quality care and safety (Shaw, 2003).

Peer Review Peer review processes are vital for maintaining clinical standards and identifying areas for improvement. They provide an opportunity for healthcare professionals to learn from each other and enhance their practice (Brennan et al., 1991).

Managing Outcome Risks

The Bottom Line The ultimate goal of managing risks is to reduce costs while improving patient outcomes. Effective risk management strategies can lead to significant cost savings by preventing errors, reducing variability, and improving efficiency (Kaplan & Mikes, 2016).

References:

1. About Financials. (2024). 18 Examples of Assets and Liabilities in Healthcare. Retrieved from https://aboutfinancials.com/examples-of-assets-and-liabilities-in-healthcare/

2. AlertMedia. (2023). Risk Management in Healthcare: From Plan to Action. Retrieved from https://www.alertmedia.com/blog/risk-management-in-healthcare/

3. ASHRM. (2024). Enterprise Risk Management: Implementing ERM. Retrieved from https://www.ashrm.org/system/files/media/file/2020/12/ERM-Implementing-ERM-for-Sucecess-White-Paper_FINAL.pdf

4. ASHRM. (2024). Professional Overview: Health Care Risk Manager. Retrieved from https://www.ashrm.org/about/hrm_overview

5. Berxi. (2024). Creating a Risk Management Plan in Healthcare [Plus Example]. Retrieved from https://www.berxi.com/resources/guides/risk-management-in-healthcare/plan/

6. Berxi. (2024). What Is Risk Management in Healthcare? Retrieved from https://www.berxi.com/resources/guides/risk-management-in-healthcare/what-it-is/

7. Brennan, T. A., Leape, L. L., Laird, N. M., Hebert, L., Localio, A. R., Lawthers, A. G., ... & Hiatt, H. H. (1991). Incidence of adverse events and negligence in hospitalized patients: Results of the Harvard Medical Practice Study I. New England Journal of Medicine, 324(6), 370-376.

8. Carroll, R. (2019). Risk management handbook for health care organizations. Jossey-Bass.

9. ECRI Institute. (2020). Patient safety and quality healthcare. ECRI Institute.

10. Ferdosi, M., Rezayatmand, R., & Molavi Taleghani, Y. (2020). Risk management in executive levels of healthcare organizations:

Insights from a scoping review. Risk Management and Healthcare Policy, 13, 215-243. https://doi.org/10.2147/RMHP.S231712

11. Ferede, Y. S., Mashwama, N. X., & Thwala, D. W. (2020). Theoretical study of the cost of poor risk management in the construction industry. ISEC Press. Retrieved from https://www.isec-society.org/ISEC_PRESS/ASEA_SEC_05/pdf/RAD-06.pdf

12. Fracttal. (2023). Maximizing Efficiency and ROI: The Importance of Asset Management in Healthcare. Retrieved from https://www.fracttal.com/en/blog/asset-management-in-healthcare

13. Grol, R., & Grimshaw, J. (2003). From best evidence to best practice: Effective implementation of change in patients' care. The Lancet, 362(9391), 1225-1230.

14. Griffith, J. R. (2020). The well-managed healthcare organization. Health Administration Press.

15. HealthcareDegree.com. (2024). Healthcare Risk Manager. Retrieved from https://www.healthcaredegree.com/administration/healthcare-risk-manager

16. HIPAA Journal. (2024). What is Risk Management in Healthcare? Retrieved from https://www.hipaajournal.com/risk-management-in-healthcare/

17. InterviewGuy. (2024). Healthcare Risk Manager Job Description. Retrieved from https://interviewguy.com/healthcare-risk-manager-job-description/

18. Jensen, R. C., et al. (2022). Risk assessment matrices: Seven attributes of risk assessment matrices. Professional Safety Journal. Retrieved from https://www.assp.org/docs/default-source/psj-articles/f1jensen_0624.pdf?sfvrsn=206346_0

19. Kaplan, R. S., & Mikes, A. (2016). Risk management—the revealing hand. Harvard Business School. Retrieved from https://www.hbs.edu/ris/Publication%20Files/16-102_397b963b-1a8b-4dcf-942f-e45acc8c9e96.pdf

20. Leape, L. L. (1994). Error in medicine. JAMA, 272(23), 1851-1857.

21. Niv, Y., & Tal, Y. (2023). Patient safety and risk management in medicine: From theory to practice. Springer. https://doi.org/10.1007/978-3-031-49865-7

22. Pittet, D., Allegranzi, B., & Storr, J. (2008). Error in medicine. American Journal of Infection Control, 36(3), 1-4.

23. Reason, J. (2000). Human error: Models and management. BMJ, 320(7237), 768-770.

24. Reason, J. (2016). Managing the risks of organizational accidents. Routledge.

25. Revnue. (2025). Why Hospitals Need Healthcare Asset Management System? Retrieved from https://revnue.com/blog/healthcare-hospital-asset-management/

26. Riskonnect. (2024). What is Healthcare Risk Management and Why Is It Important? Retrieved from https://riskonnect.com/healthcare/healthcare-risk-management/

27. Rotter, T., Kinsman, L., James, E., Machotta, A., Gothe, H., Willis, J., & Kugler, J. (2010). Clinical pathways: Effects on professional practice, patient outcomes, length of stay and hospital costs. Cochrane Database of Systematic Reviews, (3).

28. SafetyCulture. (2023). Risk Management for Healthcare Organizations. Retrieved from https://safetyculture.com/topics/risk-management/risk-management-for-healthcare/

29. Shaw, C. D. (2003). How can hospital performance be measured and monitored? World Health Organization. Retrieved from https://www.euro.who.int/__data/assets/pdf_file/0009/74718/E82975.pdf

30. Swisher, J. D., Scherer, J., & Yin, R. K. (2004). Cost-benefit estimates in prevention research. Journal of Primary Prevention, 25, 137-148. Retrieved from

https://link.springer.com/article/10.1023/B:JOPP.0000042386
.32377.c0

31. The Knowledge Academy. (2024). Hazard vs Risk: What's the Difference? Retrieved from https://www.theknowledgeacademy.com/blog/hazard-vs-risk/

32. Vincent, C. (2010). Patient safety. Wiley-Blackwell.

33. Woolf, S. H., Grol, R., Hutchinson, A., Eccles, M., & Grimshaw, J. (1999). Potential benefits, limitations, and harms of clinical guidelines. BMJ, 318(7182), 527-530.

34. Worksafe UK. (2024). The Difference Between Hazard and Risk: What You Need to Know. Retrieved from https://www.worksafe.uk.com/risk-assessment/hazard-vs-risk-whats-the-difference/

35. Youngberg, B. J. (2011). Principles of risk management and patient safety. Jones & Bartlett Learning.